Authors **Lucy Cooke** and **Laura Webber** are psychologists specialising in children's eating behaviour. They met at the Health Behaviour Research Centre at University College London and discovered a mutual interest in the development of children's food preferences and eating behaviour. Together they developed and tested techniques aimed at helping parents and carers of young children to foster healthy eating habits in their children, and to take the worry and stress out of mealtimes. More recently, Lucy has been collaborating with Great Ormond Street Hospital's Feeding and Eating Disorders Service to investigate whether these feeding techniques have application in clinical practice, while Laura has been working with the National Institute for Clinical Excellence to develop childhood weight management guidelines.

With nearly twenty years' research experience with many hundreds of children, and nearly seventy published academic papers and reports between them, Lucy and Laura have decided to bring their scientific expertise to a wider audience. Both live in London, and Lucy has two grown-up daughters who always eat their greens!

Other titles

STRESS-FREE FEEDING

Lucy Cooke and Laura Webber

ROBINSON

ROBINSON

First published in Great Britain in 2015 by Robinson

ISBN: 978-1-84528-605-7 (paperback)
ISBN: 978-1-47211-980-3 (ebook)

Typeset in Great Britain by Penny Mills
Printed and bound in Great Britain by Clays Ltd, St Ives plc
Papers used by Robinson are from well-managed forests
and other responsible sources

Robinson
is an imprint of
Constable & Robinson Ltd
Carmelite House
50 Victoria Embankment
London EC4Y 0DZ

An Hachette UK Company
www.hachette.co.uk

www.littlebrown.co.uk

This book is dedicated to
Professor Jane Wardle,
whose enormous contribution to our
understanding of child eating behaviour has
been an inspiration to us both.

CONTENTS

Acknowledgements

We are indebted to all of the parents and children who have participated in the studies described in this book, and in particular to Kate Birch, Catriona Daley, Alison Gahagan, Pippa Lally, Rebecca Webber, Samantha Baker, Chloe Livermore, Stephanie Coughlin, Amy James, Martin Brown, Heather Northridge and Jane Daley for contributing their feeding experiences. Names have been changed in the text.

In drafting this book we owe our gratitude to Jane Landon, Jennifer Saxton, Catriona Daley, Robin Ireland, Matthew Philpott, and Sarah Briggs for their perspicacious comments and to Belinda Jones for editing the manuscript.

And to our families . . .

Lucy: Love and gratitude to my husband, Simon, and to my daughters, Phoebe and Georgia, for their support, encouragement and unshakeable belief in me.

Laura: Sincere thanks to my family and friends for their support of yet another endeavour. A special thank you to Lucy with whom it has been such a pleasure and privilege to work with again.

Foreword

IF YOU ARE READING this book, you are most likely to be a parent or carer of a young child; in particular, someone who is trying to get things as right as possible in terms of setting your child up for a happy and healthy future. Nurturing and providing for offspring is, after all, a basic human instinct. In eras gone by this would have been a more straightforward matter – you breastfed your baby, foraged or hunted near to where you lived, then prepared a limited range of geographically or seasonally available edible vegetable or animal matter to feed your infant. It is interesting to speculate whether there would have been discussion and disagreement about the 'right' way to wean babies onto solids, or what foods to offer when, even when there was such limited choice. I suspect there might well have been, but I am certain it would not have been anywhere near as confusing as it is in the first part of the twenty-first century. As parents and carers, we are bombarded with opinions, advice, guidelines and a bewildering array of products all aimed at doing the thing we most want to do: feed our children in the best possible way. The problem is that so often it is impossible to negotiate all the conflicting recommendations and statements and we are left overwhelmed and uncertain rather than in a position to make confident, well-informed choices. This is precisely where this gem of a book comes in.

Simply put, the authors of this book – Lucy Cooke and Laura Webber – know what they are talking about. They are both experts in the field of feeding and eating behaviour in early childhood. They have a scientific understanding and detailed knowledge of how children's behaviour is modelled and can be shaped, in particular in relation to helping children accept a wide range of foods. They have read hundreds of publications on the subject and conducted studies of their own to help us better understand the development of healthy eating behaviour in young children. In this book they set out their synthesis of up-to-date knowledge derived from a large amount of research data in clear and accessible language. This book is *not* for you if you want to read about a shiny new approach to feeding your child. It *is* for you if you want a no-nonsense overview of research findings from studies conducted over many years in many different countries, distilled into clear information about what we do and do not know and translated into practical guidance and recommendations.

Stress-Free Feeding is a unique and empowering book. Reading it will allow parents and carers to be in a position to make informed choices and decisions about how to approach their child's feeding. The writing is authoritative and the content is reliable. Controversial topics such as television watching while eating and preparing separate types of food for children are addressed, not from a position of opinion but from one based on scientific investigation. Suggestions on how to have fun with your child as you help them develop healthy eating habits are included throughout.

Good nutrition in childhood is fundamental to health and well-being throughout life. Ensuring your child develops the appropriate behaviours to achieve good nutrition is an important responsibility for all parents and carers. With the help of this useful book your understanding of what is important will be improved, you will be able to make informed decisions and choose to apply strategies that have been demonstrated to be effective. Above all, the authors allow you to feel confident about your choices and help you to have fun feeding your child.

Dr Rachel Bryant-Waugh
Consultant Clinical Psychologist
Feeding and Eating Disorders Service
Great Ormond Street Hospital for Children
NHS Foundation Trust

Introduction

Why write this book and who is it for?

For decades, psychologists and nutritionists have been researching and testing the best ways to encourage children to eat a healthy diet. Some of the knowledge gained has made it into the public domain, but many potentially useful techniques are still unknown or misunderstood by the public as a whole. The problem is that sometimes scientists aren't brilliant at spreading the word beyond their academic peers: important findings are written up and published, but only in academic journals that are read by a tiny percentage of the population. Another problem is the scientific jargon used – even if parents do get access to the published research, it can be very hard to work out the practical application of the findings.

This book is designed to help parents and caregivers to understand how their child's food preferences and eating habits develop, and how to help them to foster a lifelong healthy relationship with food. Our aim is to translate the hard science into a digestible form (pun intended!), provide practical solutions to the most problematic and anxiety-provoking aspects of feeding children and, we hope, dispel some of the unhelpful myths and misperceptions along the way.

This is a practical guide to feeding problems and how to solve them.[1] It is not a recipe book since there are plenty of those, nor is it about nutrition as such. We are psychologists, and our expertise is in behaviour – the *how* of feeding, rather than the *what*.

Who are we?

We are psychologists by background, both having specialised for our PhD studies in children's eating behaviour. We met whilst working at the Health Behaviour Research Centre at University College London and discovered our mutual interest in the development of children's food preferences and eating habits. Together, we developed and tested techniques aimed at helping parents and carers of young children to foster healthy eating habits and to take the worry and stress out of mealtimes. We have experience of collaborating with Great Ormond Street Hospital's Feeding and Eating Disorders Service to investigate

---

[1] If your child's feeding problem is causing weight loss or excessive weight gain, social isolation, or genuine nutritional deficiency, consult your GP in the first instance.

whether these feeding techniques can be used in clinical practice, and have been working with the National Institute for Clinical Excellence to develop childhood weight management guidelines. With nearly twenty years' research experience with many hundreds of children, and nearly seventy published academic papers between us, we have decided to bring our scientific knowledge to a wider audience.

Definitions and language

We have tried to avoid jargon where possible and to be as clear as possible. Where it wasn't possible to put a concept into plain words, we hope we have explained it thoroughly.

When talking about babies and children we have sometimes used 'he' and 'him' and sometimes 'she' and 'her' because 'they' and 'their' feels clumsy. Also, we mostly talk about parents or mothers, but this is shorthand – of course we want to include mothers, fathers, grandparents, nannies, childminders, nursery teachers or anyone else who might be in charge of feeding a young child. We hope this book is relevant and useful for all of you.

How is the book organised?

Using case studies and real-life examples, this book is full of simple, practical advice on child feeding that actually works to develop healthy eating patterns for life. We start by describing what is known about the nature and nurture of children's likes and dislikes of food, and their eating habits. We go on to describe the sorts of techniques that have emerged from the scientific research as effective ways to get children eating better, healthier diets; from the milk-feeding period to around the age of five. We have included a couple of chapters aimed at helping you to sort fact from fiction in the claims made for children's foods and to make you a truly informed consumer. Finally, we have included a list of resources and sources of more information for the really keen amongst you.

This is not necessarily a book to read from start to finish: you will probably dip in and out of it for information relevant to the stage your child is currently at. What we hope is that you will come back to it when you need it, making it a useful resource for years to come.

Bon appétit!

CHAPTER ONE

Children's eating habits: nature or nurture?

ALL CHILDREN ARE DIFFERENT – their eating habits and the foods that they like and dislike differ even between siblings. You may have one child who only likes fruit and rejects vegetables, and another who is just the opposite; one of your children might eat like a horse, where another child eats almost nothing. This is baffling to parents, because most tell us that they approach feeding their children in exactly the same way. So are children born with certain likes and dislikes, or do they learn them? Are children born fussy eaters or do they become fussy because of poor parenting practices?

This chapter describes what is known about the different contribution that genes and environment make to children's food preferences and eating habits.

INNATE TASTE PREFERENCES

While each child's individual food preferences and attitudes to eating are unique, some taste preferences are innate. By innate, we mean that *all* infants are born with them. Even at birth, it is clear from their facial expressions and physical responses that babies really like sweet tastes, and really dislike sour and bitter ones. Try giving just a drop of sugar syrup and then a drop of lemon juice to a newborn and spot the difference!

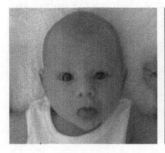 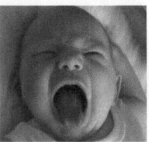

Photos © Lucy Stirling

Tasting sugar   *Tasting lemon juice*

Liking for salty flavours also appears to be universal, although it doesn't usually appear until around 3–4 months of age. Interestingly, babies born to mothers who had relatively severe morning sickness (and thus experienced low salt levels themselves) seem to be particularly keen on salty tastes.

Throughout childhood and until mid-adolescence, liking for sweet tastes is higher than in adults. In fact, the effect of sweetness is so powerful in very young children that it can actually act as a painkiller – in an American study, children were able to keep their hand in very cold water for longer when tasting a sweet substance.

Evolutionary psychologists have an intriguing explanation for the origin of these preferences. In our ancient past, when we foraged for food to eat, sweetness would have acted as a signal of the presence of useful and nutritious calories, while sour and bitter tastes might suggest the presence of harmful toxins, and thus these innate preferences would have had a useful protective purpose. No one is quite sure why we are predisposed to like salty tastes, except that sodium is something that the body needs.

GENETIC FOOD PREFERENCES

So, liking of sweet tastes (and, to a great extent, salty tastes) is common to all babies, but where do differences in food preferences between children come from? Perhaps surprisingly, quite a large contribution is made by genetic factors. That is, children inherit their parents' preferences to quite a large extent. In fact, in a recent 'nature versus nurture' investigation into food likes and dislikes, genes were found to be roughly 50 per cent responsible for differences between children's tastes. Put simply, if you hate vegetables then there's a pretty good chance that your child will too. However, unlike eye colour, which is 100 per cent determined by genes, food preferences *can* be changed. Chapter 4 will show you how.

EATING BEHAVIOUR

As well as differences in their food likes and dislikes, children vary in their attitudes to eating and behaviours around food. Psychologists working in the area of child feeding have identified a number of eating-behaviour traits that distinguish between enthusiastic and more reluctant eaters. These can be divided into what scientists have termed 'food approach' (i.e. enthusiastic) and 'food avoidant' (i.e. fussy or picky) behaviours. These are defined as follows:

Food approach

- **Food responsiveness:** the tendency to eat anything placed in front of you, regardless of whether you are hungry or not. These children are always ready to eat.

- **Enjoyment of food:** the tendency to see eating as a pleasure and to look forward to mealtimes.

- **Emotional eating:** seeking food as comfort, entertainment or to relieve boredom.

Food avoidant

- **Satiety responsiveness:** the tendency to get full up quickly. These children will rarely finish everything on their plate.

- **Food fussiness:** the rejection of new food or certain types of familiar food, resulting in a very limited diet.

- **Emotional under-eating:** the tendency to go off food when upset.

Perhaps not surprisingly, children who display more 'food approach' behaviour traits are on average heavier than those who are more 'food avoidant'.

GENETIC INFLUENCES ON EATING BEHAVIOUR

Like food preferences, eating-behaviour traits are inherited to a large extent. If parents are slow or reluctant eaters, there's a reasonable chance that their children will be likewise, although the way that genes get mixed up at conception means that you can end up with one child who is a food responsive 'plate-clearer' and one who is a satiety responsive under-eater. Here are some comments from some of our research participants:

'*She's always been a picky eater compared to her brother, who will eat anything.*'

'*I think children do vary a lot within families. If I was going to have another child now, I wouldn't assume that they were going to be the same. I think parents have a certain amount of influence but children are so different.*'

By now, we hope you will be feeling reassured that your child's idiosyncratic eating habits are not entirely the result of something you have done or failed to do. We may however have convinced you that it's all in their genes and there's nothing you can do to change things. On the contrary, although genetic factors do partly determine differences between children, so do environmental factors, by which we mean anything from the proximity of the local sweet shop to the presence of a bowl of fruit on your kitchen table; from the amount of TV your child watches to whether you eat meals together as a family. For very young children, though, the most important environmental factors are the family and the home, and these begin to exert an influence from the very earliest stages of life.

ENVIRONMENTAL INFLUENCES ON EATING BEHAVIOUR

In the womb

Towards the end of the third trimester, babies swallow as much as 400 ml of amniotic fluid daily and are thus exposed to the flavours of their mother's diet – good and bad. Not all flavours transmit but some that do are mint, garlic, carrot and caraway. In an early study in this area, researchers asked a group of pregnant women to drink carrot juice in the third trimester of their pregnancy, another group to drink it during the first three months of breastfeeding and a third to avoid carrots at both time points. When weaning their infants at 4–6 months, the babies whose mums had had the carrot juice either during pregnancy or while breastfeeding ate more carrot than those whose mums had no carrots. This suggests that eating plenty of fruit and vegetables in pregnancy might be a very effective strategy to improve children's intake of these foods in later childhood. This is good news, as long as the mother's diet is a healthy one, but there is also evidence from animal studies to suggest that a high-fat, high-sugar diet in pregnancy may predispose offspring to prefer these sorts of foods.

During milk feeding

This experience continues post-natally for breastfed babies who continue to be exposed to a variety of flavours transmitted through breast milk. If a mother's diet is rich in fruit and vegetables, this appears to increase their baby's liking for these foods in later childhood. This varied taste experience contrasts with that of formula-fed infants, who typically receive the same flavour at every mealtime and may explain why children who were breastfed tend to be less fussy than their formula-fed counterparts. Chapter 2 will cover the milk-feeding period in more detail.

At weaning

The first foods offered at the stage of introducing solids may also be influential on food preferences and eating behaviours in the long-term. Some scientists believe that there is a window of opportunity between 4 and 7 months when babies are especially receptive to new tastes and that this might be a great time to introduce less intrinsically likeable foods, such as vegetables. Certainly there is growing evidence to suggest that giving as wide a variety of tastes as possible at the early stages of weaning may reduce fussiness and promote greater acceptance of diverse foods in later childhood. Weaning is discussed in depth in Chapter 3.

FUSSY EATERS AND FOOD AVOIDERS

In the second year of life, many children who were previously enthusiastic eaters suddenly start to refuse unfamiliar foods or certain types of foods – frustratingly, it is usually fruit and vegetables that are rejected rather than sweets and cakes! This is a normal developmental stage that a large number of children go through and there is no need for serious concern.[2] Having said this, research has revealed a number of effective strategies to help parents to deal with fussy eating and to get their child back to a healthy eating routine. Chapter 4 will describe these in full.

PLATE-CLEARERS AND OVER-EATERS

Some children are almost the opposite of fussy: they seem to be hungry all the time, may eat very quickly and ask for seconds before everyone else is halfway through their meal. You may worry about their future weight, even if they appear to be about right for their age now.

---

[2] If the fussiness is accompanied by noticeable weight loss, significant nutritional deficiency and/or disruption to social relationships, seek the help of your GP in the first instance.

It will not have escaped your notice that we are experiencing a veritable epidemic of childhood obesity, and while there are a great many complex reasons for this, there are things you can do to make sure your child stays within a healthy weight range. Chapter 5 will present the latest research on the feeding practices that help to foster and nurture your child's ability to recognise and act upon their feelings of fullness or hunger.

OUTSIDE INFLUENCES

From spoiling grandparents to supermarkets, TV advertising and other media, many different forces can act to undermine and undo all your good work to get your child to eat a healthy diet. Chapters 6–8 will take on these in turn and arm you with some practical strategies to minimise the damage.

OUR PERSPECTIVE

All children are different – some are a dream to feed and others a nightmare. We know that all parents and caregivers want the best for their children and would do anything to create happy mealtimes where everyone enjoys their food and no one eats too much or too little.

While it is easier said than done in many cases, what

we hope to do is to help you to be responsive feeders from the word go: sensitive to the verbal and non-verbal signals of your child, and responding appropriately. This doesn't mean always complying with the child's request, but at least acknowledging it; it means permitting your child some autonomy over their eating, but not so much that they eat nothing but sweets; and being relaxed if things get messy when self-feeding starts – but drawing a firm line at throwing food.

Some suggestions for promoting happy mealtimes

- Be close when feeding your child – use touch and eye contact.
- Try to identify your baby's signals for hunger as distinct from tiredness, pain or discomfort.
- Respond to your baby's attention to their food – name what they point at.
- Talk at mealtimes – not just about food.
- Offer plenty of variety.
- Have a routine of meals and snack times.
- Encourage self-feeding – try to put up with the mess.
- Respect food preferences within reason – everyone dislikes some foods.
- Never force a child to eat when she says she's had enough.

CHAPTER TWO

The first six months:
milk feeding

CURRENT RECOMMENDATIONS FROM THE World Health Organization (WHO) are for exclusive breastfeeding for the first 6 months of life and, indeed, it seems that the overwhelming majority of mums want to try breastfeeding. In the UK, a massive 81 per cent of mothers start breastfeeding soon after birth, but 3 months later that figure is down to 17 per cent, and only 1 per cent of mothers manage to breast-feed exclusively until their baby is 6 months old. Although some may never have intended to breastfeed for more than a week or two, many more are clearly having sufficient difficulty that they have to give up early. This is a particularly emotive area, and some mothers who do not manage to breastfeed feel guilty, as if they have failed their babies. What is really important is that however you choose to feed your baby, you get the support you need.

Caitlin
mum of Tim (10), Lily (8) and George (4)

'If you can't do it or you're not producing enough milk or not even enjoying it, you can feel really down. Not just guilty, but also useless, especially when so many other mothers seem to be doing it well.'

This chapter will examine the science behind the recommendations, helping you to make up your own mind for what is right for you and your baby.

MAKING THE CHOICE: BREAST OR BOTTLE?

Many of the arguments in favour of breastfeeding are very well known. First and foremost, the antibodies that babies get from breast milk boost their immunity so that they are less likely to get infections than the babies fed with formula milk. They are also less likely to suffer from constipation or gastroenteritis and diarrhoea. It appears that the protective effect of breastfeeding continues into childhood too, with children who have been breastfed having a lower risk of chest and ear infections.

17

From the mum's point of view, there are lots of other advantages. For example:

- There's no sterilising of bottles, and milk at the right temperature is on tap 24 hours a day!
- It's free – formula currently costs up to £50 per month.
- It aids attachment and bonding in the early days.
- Breastfeeding helps to delay the return of your menstrual cycle.
- It burns about 500 calories a day so it helps with weight loss.
- It lowers your lifetime risk of ovarian and breast cancer.
- It speeds up your physical recovery from giving birth.

There are a number of other advantages to breast-feeding that are less well known but just as compelling. As discussed already, scientific research has revealed that breast milk carries a variety of flavours from the maternal diet and that this can affect babies' food acceptance later on – remember the carrot juice study described earlier? This experience of different flavours may be the reason for the finding that breastfed children eat more fruit and vegetables than those who were formula-fed and tend to be less fussy. There is also some evidence that breastfed babies are less likely to become overweight or to contract type-2 diabetes, high blood pressure and high cholesterol in adulthood than formula-fed babies. Scientists aren't sure why this is, but it may partly be because breast-fed babies have more control over the amount of milk that they consume. Bottle-fed babies are often encouraged to finish the bottle at every feed, even if they are showing signs of having had enough. Because breastfeeding mums can't see how much milk their baby is getting, they seem to be less likely to over-feed and more likely to let their baby decide when he has had enough.

Taken together, these make a very strong case for at least trying breastfeeding and, as we have noted, the vast majority of mothers do try soon after birth, even if many are unable or unwilling to continue for the recommended 6 months.

Some of the most common reasons given for not trying breastfeeding or for giving up early are as follows:

- 'I don't know how much she is getting.'
- 'I don't think I'm making enough milk to satisfy him.'
- 'I got mastitis and it's really painful.'
- 'My partner wants to help with some feeds.'

- 'I get embarrassed breastfeeding in public.'
- 'I need to go back to work and expressing milk is really difficult and takes ages.'

However, the overwhelming majority give up breast-feeding because they find it so much more difficult than they expected and they don't get enough support or encouragement from those around them. Many find it extremely painful at first, and not all babies seem to be terribly good at latching on.

Here are the sorts of things that mums have told us:

Diane
mum of Joshua (10 months)

'As a first-time mum, I was shocked to discover that breastfeeding wasn't easy. I had assumed it would be natural and that me and my baby would get it straight away. When we didn't, it really knocked my confidence. People should warn you.'

Carole
mum of Jordan (3) and Kai (6 months)

'For expectant mothers, I think everyone paints a rosy picture of breastfeeding, but the reality is quite different and no one likes to talk about the negatives. It's a shame, because being open about the issues women have might help more women succeed.'

Breastfeeding is something that you and your baby need to learn how to do and that takes time, patience and lots of support from family, friends and health professionals. If you are struggling but want to keep going, there are plenty of sources of information and support out there, so seek it out if you need it (see 'Resources and sources of further information' at the end of this book).

Here's someone who finally found the light at the end of the tunnel:

Alice,
mum of Nick (16 months)

'It took around 4 to 6 weeks to really get breast-feeding established – much longer than the books suggested. I wasn't surprised by how hard it was because my elder sister had really struggled with breastfeeding and had had to give up in the end. In the early weeks it was very difficult and painful, but I was really keen to do it so I persevered. Once everything had settled down, I kept thinking how much harder bottle-feeding looked – all that sterilising and making up feeds and stuff...'

SO WHAT'S WRONG WITH FORMULA-FEEDING?

The way that the guidelines are written suggests that there is no other way to feed a baby than breastfeeding:

'Infants should be exclusively breastfed – i.e. receive only breast milk – for the first 6 months of life to achieve optimal growth, development and health. "Exclusive breastfeeding" is defined as giving no other food or drink – not even water – except breast milk.'[3]

---

[3] WHO: www.who.int/elena/titles/exclusive_breastfeeding/en/

It is far from clear whether these guidelines can also be applied to formula-fed babies. That is, where the guidelines say exclusive *breast*feeding for 6 months, should they actually say "exclusive milk-feeding" or are the recommendations for formula-fed babies different? If so, what are those recommendations? In fact, exactly the same rules probably apply to formula-fed babies, but it seems as though there is a belief that by even mentioning infant formula, the WHO might be seen as encouraging its use and discouraging breastfeeding.

This issue needs to be placed in context. The fact is that in under-developed and low-income countries, there have been accusations of foul play against the baby-milk manufacturers. They have been accused of using tactics to undermine breastfeeding and promote formula-feeding, even where the water supply is not safe and facilities for sterilising are non-existent. As a result, some pressure groups maintain, many infants have died unnecessarily and therefore there is ongoing monitoring of the practices of manufacturers in these regions. Obviously, in the developed world, facilities and standards of hygiene are vastly better and safer, running water is literally on tap! This means that formula-feeding in Western countries is what the WHO has termed 'AFASS' – acceptable, feasible, affordable, sustainable and safe, albeit that they also maintain that 'breast is best'.

Understandably, feelings run high around this topic, but it is beyond the scope or aim of this book to enter further into the debate. It's our belief that mothers want to do the best they can for their babies, but have to compromise sometimes for their own sanity!

Alice
mum of Nick (16 months)

'I had a lot of support to keep going from friends who had been through it all before. One older friend in particular was the voice of reason and made me realise that it wasn't the end of the world if he had a small amount of formula every once in a while.'

From here on in this chapter, the advice provided will be aimed at both breast- and formula-feeding mums, as most of the scientific findings can be applied to both.

THE FIRST SIX MONTHS: MILK FEEDING

FEEDING ON DEMAND OR ON SCHEDULE?

The frequency with which babies want to be fed varies enormously, and they also vary in the efficiency of their feeding technique. Some babies have an avid sucking style that empties a breast in no time at all, whereas others stop and start, or are easily distracted, so that every feed takes an hour or more. As we said in Chapter 1 every baby is different and, in the first few weeks, there may be no apparent pattern to your baby's feeding needs, but gradually you will establish a routine that suits you both.

There is considerable debate on whether it is best to feed on demand or whether it is better to try to establish a schedule. A number of popular childcare books advocate a strict timetable of feeding and sleeping, 'from day one, so that you avoid months of sleepless nights, colic, excessive crying, feeding difficulties and many other problems that we are so often told are a normal part of parenting'.[4]

This is another area where feelings get very heated, with both demand- and schedule-feeders claiming the best outcomes for babies. A recent study of over 10,000 babies in the UK looked at differences in school

---

[4] www.contentedbaby.com/gina.htm

achievement between children who, as infants, had been fed on demand and those who had been fed on schedule. The study showed that babies who were fed when they were hungry – with breast milk or formula – achieved higher scores in SAT[5] tests at ages 5, 7, 11 and 14, and that by the age of 8 they had an IQ 4–5 points higher. However, mothers who keep to a schedule seem to be happier, scoring higher on well-being measures and reporting feeling more confident and less tearful – presumably because they feel more in control.

There would, therefore, appear to be a trade-off between cognitive benefits to the baby in terms of mental development, and emotional benefits to mums! Although the sheer number of participants in this study is impressive, these are early findings and need to be replicated before any real conclusions are drawn. Just because there were differences in IQ between demand- and schedule-fed babies does not mean that these differences were *caused* by the choice of feeding method. On balance, though, it makes sense to allow a degree of flexibility in feeding and to try to be sensitive and responsive to your baby's attempts at communicating their needs.

---

[5] Standardised Assessment Tests used in UK schools.

DREAM FEEDING: THE WAY TO A GOOD NIGHT'S SLEEP?

Precisely the opposite of responding to your baby's needs, 'dream feeding' is nevertheless growing in popularity. Also known as 'focal feeds', 'top-up feeds' or 'rollover feeds', dream feeds involve feeding your infant just before you go to bed, without waking him. The idea is that this will fill him up and make him sleep for longer so that you get more rest. Despite its popularity, there has been very little research (two published studies to date) to show if dream feeds are effective for helping with sleep, or whether they have any adverse effects. Success stories are mainly anecdotal, with some parents swearing by them and others saying it did not work for them, or made things worse! However, of the two published studies of dream feeding, both found an increase in sleep time in infants receiving a 'focal feed'. But again, it is what works best for you and your baby that matters.

If you decide to try it, this is how to do it:

- Just before you go to bed, between 10 p.m. and 11 p.m., gently pick up your baby, without making any loud noises and without turning the light on.

- To get a sleepy baby to start feeding, stroke his cheek to start the rooting reflex[6].

- Give as long a feed as you can without fully waking your baby.

- Put him back down to sleep.

Obviously, this can be done whether you are breast- or bottle-feeding and can be done by a partner or relative if you make up a bottle or express some breast milk. A word of warning, though: scientists have revealed that the composition of breast milk varies over the course of a day and that only milk expressed at night should be fed to babies at night. Milk expressed in the morning may actually wake your baby up!

There are also some possible downsides to this practice that you need to consider:

- At this time of night, babies are typically very deeply asleep so it may be very difficult to rouse them enough to feed them. Obviously you shouldn't feed a baby who is lying down because of the risk of choking.

---

[6] A rooting reflex is a reflex that is seen in newborn babies, who automatically turn the face toward the food and make sucking (rooting) motions with the mouth when the cheek or lip is touched. The rooting reflex helps to ensure successful breastfeeding.

- You are interfering with your baby's natural sleeping/waking cycle and this may mean that he actually wakes more rather than less often in the end.

- You may be setting up a night-feeding routine that wouldn't have occurred naturally.

In the absence of any convincing evidence either for or against dream feeding, we'll leave it to you to decide if it's right for you and your baby.

Kate
mum of Ben (18 months)

'I used dream feeding in the hope that he would sleep on longer. One bottle at 11 p.m. Then I went cold turkey one night and just stopped it and it didn't make any difference to what time he woke. Most people I know did it. One friend didn't stop and is still doing it at 18 months – I think some babies start to rely on it, wake up for it and expect it so she's created a need.'

Jen
mum of Maddy (14 months)

'I didn't dream feed. It just didn't seem in line with the baby's natural rhythm.'

A COMPROMISE: RESPONSIVE FEEDING

There is growing interest in what has been termed 'responsive parenting'. The idea is that mothers need to communicate with their babies, and to notice and respond to their baby's attempts to communicate back. Obviously it takes time to learn how to interpret each other's behaviour accurately, but babies are surprisingly good communicators, even in their first hours and days of life. Within an hour of being born they can imitate facial expressions and within 15 hours they are able to recognise their mum's voice and prefer their mum's face to others.

When it comes to communication around feeding, mums need to learn to recognise when their infant is hungry and to feed them promptly, and then to stop when the baby signals that he is full. Signs of fullness might be turning the head away or sucking much more slowly, although it can be quite hard to tell in the early days. As time goes on, however, mums learn to distinguish their baby's hungry cry from a tired or bored cry and can act accordingly. This way, it is claimed, infants develop the ability to self-regulate their intake – in other words, to eat when hungry and stop when they are full.

Feeding a baby when it is not hungry (for example, encouraging a baby to finish a bottle when he seems to have had enough) overrides this ability and it is thought to be associated with a higher risk of being overweight in later life. Try to remember that your baby's stomach is tiny – about the size of his closed fist – and he will get full up more quickly than you think.

MORE THAN JUST FOOD

Of course feeding is not only about the food – it also offers the opportunity to establish a close attachment between mother and baby. Gentle, affectionate touching and lots of mother–child eye-contact while feeding is vitally important and seems to protect against later feeding difficulties, to some extent. Whilst breastfeeding obviously affords more opportunity for close contact, looking into infants' faces whilst bottle-feeding also encourages intake, so however you feed your baby, try to make it an interaction between the two of you rather than something you are imposing on him.

TAKE-HOME MESSAGES

We all know that 'breast is best' – even the infant-formula manufacturers can't claim otherwise – but not everyone can manage it, some don't want to and some are forced to give up early for a variety of reasons such as work commitments or infection. However you choose to feed your baby, make sure it's YOUR choice and, if you are having difficulty with breastfeeding but want to keep going, shout for help from anyone you can get your hands on. There is loads of evidence that the people who manage to master breastfeeding are those who receive the most help and support from friends, relatives and health professionals. This is because breastfeeding isn't easy for everyone, whatever they tell you. What *is* true is that many people regret not breastfeeding, but very few regret that they did.

- The evidence in favour of breastfeeding is overwhelming, not just for your baby but for you, too – give it your best shot!

- Bear in mind that it will take a while to get it working perfectly – don't give up too soon.

TAKE-HOME MESSAGES

- If you really can't breastfeed or if you simply don't want to, don't feel guilty – your baby will be fine.

- However you decide to feed your baby, give lots of cuddles, stroking and eye-contact whilst doing it.

- Try to distinguish between different cries and respond accordingly.

- Don't make your baby finish the bottle if he seems to have had enough.

CHAPTER THREE

Weaning:
the transition to solid food

THE INTRODUCTION OF FOODS other than milk is an
exciting time for both mothers and babies, but it can
also be an anxiety-provoking time, not least because
advice from health organisations, health professionals,
relatives and friends is often contradictory and, as
with breastfeeding, opinions are strongly held and
sometimes aggressively defended. In this chapter,
we will discuss the when, what and how of weaning,
comparing official recommendations with what
actually happens in practice. We will also discuss the
current understanding of the importance of weaning
in the development of lifelong food preferences and
eating habits.

WHEN TO WEAN?

Babies will continue to rely on milk (either breast
or first formula) as the prime source of calories and
nourishment for most of their first year of life. However,
after this time they start to need additional nutrients,

particularly iron, and it is generally accepted that complementary foods should start to be offered no later than 6 months of age. The World Health Organization recommends exclusive milk feeding until this age and official guidelines in many countries echo this, although there is general acceptance that mothers can and do begin to introduce solids before 6 months. This is a controversial area, but it is our belief that all infants are different and it makes little sense to be inflexible when mothers are quite capable of recognising when their own child is ready for more than milk alone.

Most agree that the signs of readiness are:

- Being able to sit up and hold their head steady.
- Having the co-ordination to look at food, pick it up and bring it to their mouths.
- Being able to swallow safely.

And that these are not signs of being ready:

- Ceasing to sleep through the night having done so previously.
- Fist chewing.
- Wanting extra milk.

Clearly, these developmental milestones will not be reached in all infants at 6 months: some may reach them earlier, while those who were born prematurely or have developmental delays develop on a very different timescale. Guidelines should be sufficiently flexible to allow for this.

What is the evidence?

The research on which the WHO guidelines were based has been questioned on the basis that most of the evidence came from developing countries or from less well-designed studies. While 6 months of exclusive breastfeeding is a sensible recommendation for reducing the spread of infection in the developing world where clean water and food may be scarce, it may have less validity in developed countries.

A window of opportunity?

Some scientists have argued that 6 months may even be a little late to begin weaning. It has been suggested that there may be a useful 'window of opportunity' to introduce babies to new tastes and flavours between the ages of 4 and 7 months. Acceptance of unfamiliar foods appears to be particularly high at this stage, and experiments have shown that whereas a toddler may need repeated experience of a food before they will consume it in reasonable quantities, 4 to 6-month-old infants will rapidly accept new flavours after very little exposure.

In a large study of over 3,000 Dutch infants, when compared with those weaning after 6 months, babies who were introduced to solid foods between 4 and 6 months enjoyed food more, but research findings have been mixed. One smaller study (less than 150 participants) found that infants weaned before 6 months were fussier feeders in later childhood, while a large-scale project looking at thousands of families in 4 European countries found very little relationship between the age of weaning and later acceptance of fruit and vegetables.

Weighing up the evidence is tricky, but it is safe to say that the results of studies of large populations give compelling evidence of an advantage in not necessarily waiting until 6 months of age.

Allergies

A further reason to consider starting weaning before 6 months concerns the development of allergies. It was originally thought that delaying introducing certain foods (for example, those containing gluten) reduced the likelihood of coeliac disease or other allergic conditions. In fact, some evidence suggests the opposite, and the European Food Safety Authority (EFSA) has recently suggested that introducing foods that contain gluten while breastfeeding might be positively beneficial in infants without a family history of coeliac disease. The EFSA goes on to state that weaning between 4 and 6 months poses no risk of adverse health outcomes, and might benefit some babies who may need additional sources of nutrients before 6 months of age.

The reality

Whatever the recommendations, in the UK, only 6 per cent of mums wait until 6 months to start introducing solids. In the USA it is 7 per cent. Clearly mothers are not adhering to official guidelines and research into the reasons for this has found that the overwhelming majority of mothers believe that milk alone has ceased to be sufficient for their baby's needs.

FIRST FOODS

Most sources of information and guidance suggest baby rice, fruit and vegetables as first foods, followed by dairy and protein foods such as yoghurt, fish and eggs with no added salt, sugar or artificial sweetener. In a recent survey, well over 50 per cent of mums offered baby rice first, perhaps because it seems pure, safe and most similar to the milk that the baby is accustomed to, and there is an assumption that a child's first solid foods should be bland. Only 8 per cent of infants are offered fruit, and only 7 per cent vegetables. This is a lost opportunity because, as we will see, research shows that babies are very receptive to new tastes and flavours and so the weaning stage might be an ideal time to introduce 'problem' foods like the less sweet, green vegetables.

Vegetables first

Despite the small numbers offering fruit and vegetables as first foods, research has repeatedly shown that the earlier in the weaning process these valuable foods are introduced, the greater the child's acceptance of them in later childhood. In Portugal, it is customary to give babies vegetable soups as their first foods – it is perhaps not surprising that Portugal has the highest intake of fruit and vegetables in Europe.

Caitlin
mum of Tim (10), Lily (8) and George (4)

'The best way I found of doing things was puréeing different types of fruit/veg, freezing in ice cube trays and then defrosting when needed. I just kept experimenting and the more tastes he tried, the more he wanted different tastes. In the same way that children's brains are sponges, so are their tastebuds.'

Misleading facial expressions

As we discussed in Chapter 1, babies are born with a preference for sweet tastes and an apparent dislike of tastes that are sour or bitter. These innate likes and dislikes can be easily seen from their facial expressions.

Later on, observing your baby grimacing at the taste of broccoli might discourage you from offering it again, but research shows that expressions can be deceptive and that despite pulling funny faces, infants may willingly continue to eat what is offered to them.

Sally
mum of Daisy (3)

'I did it when she was about 4 to 5 months old. Started with a baby cereal mixed with hot water. Used the smallest amounts at the beginning and gradually built up the quantity and then started introducing new foods. Mashed banana, avocado, stewed apples and all different sorts of veg. Carrot was the first veg and I can remember seeing Daisy's face at first taste was a 'What the hell is this?' and then she liked it.'

This is very important, as some of the best and most healthy foods to offer an infant are not sweet, like the milk they are used to. It appears that the faces they make indicate surprise at an unfamiliar taste rather than an aversion, so it's worth focusing on what they are eating rather than whether they actually look as though they are enjoying it. Babies will look happier in response to sweeter foods and this can lead mums to try to sweeten vegetable purées by mixing them with sweeter fruit purées. Results suggest that this is unnecessary and may even be counterproductive.

Facial expressions of apparent dislike should not be confused with genuine rejection – indicated by spitting out, clamping the mouth shut and turning the head away. It's probably best to give up for the day if you get these sorts of reactions.

Keep going

However, even foods that have been completely rejected once or twice may come to be enjoyed after a few more attempts, according to a large body of research from the USA and the UK. Rejection of vegetables in particular is not uncommon in infants, but after up to 8 or so tastings, most foods are accepted.

Offer lots of variety

However, there needs to be a balance between persistence and overkill. Recently, researchers have begun to focus on the importance of variety in the first foods offered to infants. Having observed an increase in liking and consumption when different foods are offered every day, we conducted a study in which mums were asked to offer 5 vegetables as first foods for the first 2 weeks of weaning, changing the vegetable they offered each day, like this:

Day 1	Day 2	Day 3	Day 4	Day 5	Day 6	Day 7
Carrot	Spinach	Peas	Swede	Parsnip	Carrot	Spinach
Day 8	Day 9	Day 10	Day 11	Day 12	Day 13	Day 14
Peas	Swede	Parsnip	Carrot	Spinach	Peas	Swede

So, babies received 2 or 3 tastes of each vegetable in total. On day 15, babies who were fed on this schedule ate much more of a completely unfamiliar artichoke purée than those who hadn't, and their mums thought they liked it more. We concluded that having the experience of lots of different tastes over the 15 days of the study made the babies more willing to eat something new. We don't know how long this effect lasts, but it certainly appears to be a promising start to a healthy and varied diet.

Caitlin
mum of Tim (10), Lily (8) and George (4)

'I was very determined at continuing to push different flavours and tastes at them all, because I wanted them, from an early age, to have a "discerning palate" and a taste for healthy but flavourful foods. I think this is part of the problem – parents are often too limited with flavours, to what they know only. Luckily, having lived overseas in countries with different flavours and ideas about feeding children – in Singapore, 1-year-olds eat raw fish and spicy broths – we too went down that path, with great results. My 4-year-old pretty much eats anything now.'

Homemade or bought?

There has been some debate about whether home-prepared foods are significantly better in any way than commercial infant foods. The laws governing the production of infant food products are stringent, meaning that they are very safe and may also contain added vitamins. However, as any grown-up who has tasted them will testify, they don't taste much like real family foods. In addition, the widespread use of fruit to sweeten many commercial baby food products leads to some bizarre combinations of ingredients: 'broccoli, pea and pear', 'plum, pear, parsnip and swede' and 'carrot, mango and banana' are good examples. These are flavours that children are unlikely to encounter in real life and may lead to the expectation that all food is sweet. It makes sense to give infants the opportunity to explore the actual flavours of individual foods – 'to develop their palate', as French mothers state they are trying to do. This is an interesting perspective on the weaning process and one, it is reasonable to speculate, not often held by UK mums.

In an ideal world, infants would be introduced to healthy, salt- and sugar-free family foods from the word go, but in practice many family diets are not this perfect and many mothers will come to rely on commercial baby foods.

We would like to offer a word of caution about commercial baby foods and the recent proliferation of pouches as the packaging method of choice for baby foods. These pouches were first developed by the organic baby-food manufacturers, but have now spread into the mainstream and are seen as aspirational and indicative of high quality. The pouches have a spout that is intended as a means of squeezing out the contents into a bowl for spoon-feeding, but it also allows babies to suck the contents out themselves, without the need for plates and spoons. While not encouraged by the manufacturers, we have anecdotal evidence that this is a common practice amongst parents when out and about. Can we make a plea here that you avoid this where possible? Sucking on a spout requires the same motor actions as sucking on a teat or a nipple, and results in the contents being delivered straight to the back of the mouth for swallowing. This is the appropriate process for dealing with liquids, but not with food. Food requires manipulation by chewing, followed by moving it from the front to the back of the mouth for swallowing – an absolutely vital lesson for babies to learn. So while the occasional meal on the go that pouches permit is fine, try to serve their contents with a spoon most of the time.

Research into the long-term effects of the types of foods offered during weaning suggests that there are multiple benefits to offering home-cooked foods rather than commercial foods. For example, in one study of over 500 infants, those who had been fed more home-cooked foods were less likely to be overweight at the age of 4 years. In a further study of nearly 8,000 children, those who had been given more home-prepared fruit and vegetables during the weaning process ate more of both at the age of 7 years, when compared with babies fed with more commercially produced foods.

PURÉES, FINGER FOODS OR BOTH?

Most guidance suggests starting babies on tiny spoonfuls of purées or mashed foods alongside soft finger foods such as cooked fruit or vegetables. However, growing interest and a great deal of heated debate has recently been forthcoming on the subject of 'baby-led weaning' (BLW). The idea is that instead of being offered bland purées, infants are seated at the family dinner table and given the same foods that the rest of the family are consuming. These foods should be in a form that they are able to pick up and bring to their mouth without assistance – large, chip-shaped pieces of soft foods roughly the size of their fist. Of course, this assumes that what the family is eating is relatively solid in texture – soup or pasta would be very challenging for a 6-month-old baby to hold in his hand! The theory is that babies will gradually, and at their own pace, learn the skills needed to get the food into their mouths and then to chew and swallow.

So far so good, but while they are learning, parents need to have a great deal of patience and a high tolerance for mess, as most of the food is likely to end up on walls and floors and very little in the baby's stomach. However, at the early stages of weaning this is not important as the baby's principal source of food should still be milk, whether breast or formula.

Penny
mum of Poppy (6) and Stan (2)

'Until Poppy was 9 months old, I religiously followed the instructions in my baby-led weaning book, so she had absolutely no purées at all. Her first meal was Christmas lunch because she had just reached 6 months of age the day before! I used to put her highchair on a large sheet of plastic to catch all the mess and she would often be naked, otherwise she would need a complete change of clothes after eating!'

Guidelines concerning both traditional and BLW approaches to weaning make the assumption that babies will be around 6 months old when offered their first foods. As discussed, we know that this is rarely the case and so deciding on the way in which foods are presented will depend on the age and motor skills of your baby. In practice, the sort of pragmatic approach taken by most health professionals is likely to be followed successfully by most parents – that is, to encourage self-feeding including offering finger foods, in parallel with spoon-feeding.

What is the evidence?

Some extravagant claims are made for baby-led weaning, including lower risk of obesity and other chronic adult conditions, higher IQ, and less pickiness in children weaned this way, but as yet no convincing evidence exists to back up these assertions.

There has been very little research on BLW, perhaps because it is very new, but also because it is not possible to conduct truly objective research in this area. A robust investigation of the effects of BLW in the short and longer term would involve randomly allocating mothers and their infants to BLW or traditional weaning groups and comparing outcomes over many years. This has not been attempted yet, and it is doubtful whether it could be achieved ethically or, indeed, whether mothers would consent to be randomly assigned to a weaning method.

Who uses BLW?

What the scant research does reveal is that the mothers who use baby-led weaning are quite different from the general population in terms of education, income, age and confidence (all are higher than average). They are also more likely to be married and to have breastfed for longer than those taking a more traditional route to weaning. When considering the logistics of BLW, the findings should not surprise us: to do it successfully, you probably need to be a stay-at-home mum, to be happy to wait until 6 months to embark upon it, you must be fearless in the face of the frequent gagging that occurs when babies encounter lumps of food for the first time, and so on.

A further concern is that one study found that the family foods that babies were being offered was higher in fat, salt and sugar and lower in iron and calories than is recommended.

Can babies eat enough with BLW?

Supporters of baby-led weaning state that babies will receive adequate nourishment from milk until 8 months of age, by which time they will have mastered the self-feeding skills necessary to consume significant amounts of food. Some research suggests that on the contrary, quite a large proportion of children are not reliably self-feeding by 8 months old, and a few won't even have begun to reach for food yet.

Penny
mum of Poppy (6) and Stan (2)

'I went on breastfeeding at the same time and so I wasn't worried about how much she was actually managing to eat, but when I went back to work when she was 9 months old, I had to express milk at work, sometimes twice during the day, and that was a bit of a nightmare. At that point, I started allowing spoons sometimes to help her to eat a bit more food.'

On balance, it seems clear that there are advantages to baby-led weaning in terms of less meal preparation, but that a combination of spoon-fed purées and finger foods is probably the most sensible approach to take and is in line with current recommendations from the Department of Health in the UK.

INTRODUCING TEXTURE – LUMPS AND BITS!

Regardless of when or how you start introducing solid foods, sometime around the seventh or eighth month your baby needs to experience foods with more texture. Finger foods are part of this process, but even spoon-fed foods should now contain soft lumps for chewing practice – mashed foods rather than purées, or added rice or pasta to provide texture. Don't worry if your baby is short of teeth: gums work perfectly well!

This is a potentially nerve-wracking period where the baby's frequent gagging may have you repeatedly practising the Heimlich manoeuvre. At this stage, raw vegetables and fruit can cause problems and raw apple and grapes are particularly common causes of gagging and even choking, so are best avoided for a little while, but the same foods cooked and roughly mashed should be fine.

Gagging can be alarming, but it is not the same as choking. In fact, gagging is a safety mechanism to *prevent* choking. In very young babies it is a highly effective and sensitive reflex and is triggered further forward in the mouth than in older children or adults, precisely in order to expel a potential problem food before it gets anywhere near their airway. Provided that your baby is sitting upright, gagging will serve to push the food forward rather than back down the throat. Saying all this, NEVER leave a small baby alone while eating.

Whatever you do, don't postpone the introduction of lumpy foods for too long. A growing body of evidence suggests that early experience with texture pays off in the long run. In an ongoing study of over 8,000 families in the Bristol area of the UK, introducing lumps into the diet after 9 months of age was associated with more feeding difficulties at 15 months and with lower fruit and vegetable intake and more feeding problems at age 7 years. As discussed in relation to taste acceptance, it may be that there is a window of opportunity for texture introduction that, if missed, can result in problems later on. Of course, the ways that these studies are carried out means that we can't say for certain that early introduction to lumps directly causes children to accept foods more readily – it may be that babies who are generally easier to feed get offered lumpy foods earlier rather than the other way around – but since there do not appear to be any negative consequences, then it probably makes sense to offer those lumpy foods as soon as your baby can cope with them.

However, there are some children who will continue to struggle with lumps and foods with certain specific textures, and others with strong flavours, colours or temperatures. This sort of sensory sensitivity may persist over time and can make feeding very difficult. In these cases, it is a good idea to see your GP and if necessary seek referral to a feeding specialist – the longer these sorts of problems are left untreated, the more difficult they are to extinguish.

By the end of your baby's first year, she will be able to eat almost anything that you do and feeding becomes simpler by the day. Try to eat together as a family as often as possible, but even if you can't manage this because of working hours and other issues, give your baby the same healthy food that you are going to eat. Remember, despite what the food industry wants us to believe, there are not adult foods and children's foods – there is just FOOD.

MILK FEEDING DURING WEANING

Fortified milks

Whether you wean traditionally using spoons and purées or whether your baby eats the same as everyone else from day one, she will continue to rely on milk for most of her nourishment in the early stages. But what kind of milk is best? In recent years, the baby-milk manufacturers have developed a range of milks known as 'follow-on' milk, and 'goodnight' milk, for babies from 6 month onwards, and 'toddler' milk or 'growing-up' milk for babies over 12 months. Typically, these milks contain less calcium and more sugar than cow's milk, although they also contain more iron and vitamin D. While the WHO suggests these milks are an unnecessary part of a baby's diet, baby-milk companies have marketed them in such a way as to imply that babies can't get the vital nutrients that they need from food and first milks alone. This sort of marketing tactic is discussed in more detail in Chapter 8, but it certainly works to sell products since these milks are the fastest-growing sector of the infant milk market.

The truth of the matter is that while your child may get some extra iron and vitamin D from follow-on milks, they also get extra sugars and proteins that may be unnecessary. If you are really concerned that your infant is getting too little iron, for instance, consult your pharmacist or GP. Vitamin drops in some water are a much better solution, since over-consumption of iron (a real risk if large quantities of these milks are being consumed) is not only unnecessary but may actually be harmful.

So should all babies be having these special milks instead of first formula or breast-milk? In a word, no. Both the World Health Organization and the Department of Health in England have concluded that infants do not need any of these, and there is NO evidence for their superiority over normal formula or breast milk, providing the baby is receiving a normal, healthy diet full of fresh vegetables, fruit and fibre. Further, unlike newborn formula milks, follow-on milks are less regulated and different varieties vary in quality.

From 6 to 12 months of age, babies should continue to receive normal formula or breast milk and, after that, they can be given full-fat cow's milk.

Sally
mum of Daisy (3)

'I never used it. One thing was that Daisy was dairy intolerant so there probably would not have been a brand that would have catered for her. The other thing is that I worked for the Department of Health in England in obesity and nutrition, and had learnt very early on that these were all a scam to convince mothers that babies need it – for companies to make money, not to help nutritionally with the baby.'

Why do these products exist?

You may now be wondering why these products exist if there is no need for them. The fact is that since 1995, advertising formula milk for babies under 6 months of age has been illegal. This regulation does not apply to milks for infants over 6 months, however. As a result, baby-milk manufacturers have invested heavily in promoting these products, resulting in substantial increases in brand awareness amongst mums and massive increases in sales (21.5 per cent growth in sales in 2010). Importantly, the packaging of these milks often strongly resembles that of their normal formula.

Be very careful not to buy one of these products by mistake if your baby is under 6 months of age, as they are not safe for this age group.

TAKE-HOME MESSAGES

It seems that there is considerable disparity between official recommendations and what mothers actually do at the stage of introducing solid foods. Even among scientists there is little consensus, but the best evidence suggests that you can't go far wrong if you follow these guidelines:

- Provided that infants are showing the signs of readiness for more than just milk, there would appear to be no harm in offering foods from 4 months onwards, although many will thrive on milk alone until around 6 months.

- Delaying complementary feeding until after 6 months may risk missing a particularly receptive stage in an infant's developing relationship with food, so offer plenty of variety straight away.

- First foods needn't be bland infant cereals – try strong-tasting vegetables like cauliflower or swede.

- As often as possible, offer home-cooked family

TAKE-HOME MESSAGES

foods rather than commercial baby foods, although remember not to add sugar or salt.

- Don't mix sweet tastes with more bitter or sour tastes – boycott the broccoli and pear combinations on offer from the food companies.

- Offer something different every day.

- Judge whether your baby has had enough by his willingness to go on eating, and NOT by his facial expression.

- Don't delay introducing foods with texture and soft lumps.

- Follow-on milks are unnecessary – continue with breast milk or first formula until age 1 year, and then introduce full-fat cow's milk.

CHAPTER FOUR

'I hate peas':
The problem of fruit and vegetables

WE ALL KNOW THAT we should try to eat at least 5 portions of fruit and vegetables (FV) a day, but very few of us manage it. On average, children in the UK eat about 3 servings daily, and adults don't do much better. But is it really important?

Well, yes it is. The vitamins, minerals and fibre that fruit and vegetables contain protect against heart disease and some cancers, and may help to maintain a healthy weight. Nevertheless, getting children to eat them is extremely difficult. Picky children are particularly at risk for low FV intake, but many enthusiastic 'plate-clearers' also have a problem with vegetables.

In this chapter, we will explain what we know about why children don't eat enough fruit and vegetables and how you can help your child to eat AND enjoy their 5 a day.

WHY DON'T CHILDREN EAT ENOUGH FRUIT AND VEGETABLES?

Generally speaking, children eat the foods that they like (or are most familiar with) and reject the ones they don't. That suggests that the reason that children don't eat enough fruit and vegetables is that they don't like them. In the case of vegetables, this would seem to be true. In a large-scale survey of over 1,500 children aged 4 to 16 years of age, we found that children of all ages liked sweet, salty and fatty foods best, and vegetables least. However, it might be a surprise to learn that fruit came a very close second to those junk foods, and when it came to individual fruits like strawberries and seedless grapes, many children said they were their favourite foods of all.

FRUIT AND FRUIT JUICE

So if children like fruit so much, how come they aren't eating enough? It makes sense for children to like fruit as it is mostly very sweet and, as we've discussed in previous chapters, they have an innate liking for sweet tastes. The explanation for low intake of fruit may lie in the context in which fruit is offered – very often in competition with sweeter, more palatable desserts or snacks. For example, how many 5-year-olds do you imagine would turn down a packet of chocolate buttons in favour of an apple? Offered a choice between a banana and a sweetened fromage frais, most children will choose the latter.

While you may like to offer your child some degree of choice in the food they eat, we believe that they are not able to make healthy choices for themselves – that's your job.

Penny
mum of Poppy (6) and Stan (2)

'I do give them some choice – I might ask them what they want to eat, but I won't necessarily give them what they say they want. I think quite carefully about the choices I give them and try to only offer a choice when I would be happy for them to have either option.'

In other words, it's better to offer the choice between a tangerine and a banana, than a tangerine and a strawberry mousse.

Another observation from our research concerns the way that parents sometimes present fruit as second best. If your mum said: 'Sorry, darling, there's no pudding today, you can have some fruit instead,' what conclusion would you draw? Clearly, Mum thinks that fruit is not nice enough to be a dessert! Children pick up on these subliminal messages, so try to say something more like, 'You're in luck today – I've got a lovely peach for your pudding.' Grown-ups can underestimate how much children regard fruit as a treat, as this mum told us:

Jill
mum of Charlotte (7) and Grace (4)

'A friend and I were organising a joint 6th birthday party for our daughters and I suggested having iced biscuits as a treat after the sandwiches and crisps and before the birthday cake. My friend insisted on seedless grapes instead. I wasn't convinced – I thought the children would leave those and just eat the cake, but I agreed in the end, and the children absolutely devoured them and asked for more.'

Niall

dad of Laura (6)

'Laura loves Fridays because she gets fish fingers at school. But she's really good, she chooses fruit rather than the pudding option for after.'

Most children need very little persuading to eat fruit as long as it's available; and again, while this sounds obvious, a full fruit bowl within view will have most children asking for it. The science backs this up. A number of studies have shown that in homes where plenty of fruit is available, children eat more of it.

Here are some more strategies that research has shown to be effective in increasing fruit intake:

- **Big it up!** Tell your child how delicious fruit is, not that it's good for them. In one study, telling children that a drink was healthy made them like it less. From a young age, they seem to think that healthy food doesn't taste as good as unhealthy food, so make sure you say how good fruit tastes. In a study at a nursery school in the USA, teachers eating mango and saying how much they liked it encouraged more children to eat it than any other tactic tried.

- **Eat it yourself:** Be a good role model. Your child wants to be like you, so if you eat plenty of fruit, they will be more likely to follow suit. Get everyone in the family on board. Role models can be dads, grandparents, siblings and friends – in fact, any individual trusted and known by the child will do.

- **Cut it up!** Most children prefer bite-sized pieces rather than the whole fruit. Fun shapes work well too.

What about fruit juice?

Fruit juice, even 100 per cent unsweetened juice, can only ever be counted as one portion of fruit in a day because it lacks the fibre content of whole fruit. In addition, the sugar in whole fruit is less damaging than in juice as it is contained within the structure of the fruit. These sugars are released when the fruit is crushed to make juice. Don't offer more than one glass of fruit juice per day, always dilute it with water and, if possible, with a meal. Try to get your child into the habit of drinking water or milk only, at other times of the day.

THE PROBLEM OF VEGETABLES

These ideas should help to increase fruit intake, but vegetables typically present more of a problem, although these techniques are certainly worth a try. Unlike fruit, vegetables are rarely sweet, and together with their low calorie content, lack of sweetness (and, in some cases, outright bitterness) means that vegetables are rejected more often than any other foods. But they are key to a healthy diet because they are packed full of natural vitamins, minerals and fibre.

Low vegetable intake is not a problem unique to UK or US children; even French children, who are often held up as good examples in this area, don't consume as many vegetables as guidelines recommend. As a consequence, a considerable amount of research (both by scientists and by the food industry) has been conducted to test different ways of making vegetables more acceptable – from cutting them into star shapes, to colouring them pink or flavouring them with chocolate. In the late nineties a popular supermarket chain developed a 'wacky veg' range, consisting of chocolate-flavoured carrots, pizza-flavoured sweetcorn, baked-bean-flavoured peas and cheese-and-onion flavoured cauliflower. These are no longer available, presumably because they didn't sell as well as anticipated.

Role modelling

As we discussed in the section on fruit, acting as a role model is one of the simplest and most powerful techniques available. Study after study has shown that if significant others (anyone important to your child – you, grandparents, siblings, friends, teachers and nannies) eat and seem to be enjoying any kind of food, then children will copy them. If you don't like or eat vegetables, or if you do eat them but show how much you dislike them by grumbling or making a face, you really can't expect your child to greet them with much enthusiasm.

If you really have a problem with vegetables, you may want to try some of the following techniques on yourself . . .!

'Exposure': the power of repeated tiny tastes

The reason that we want children to like vegetables as well as eat them is that then they will go on eating them in the future. What we know is that familiarity leads to liking, and liking leads to eating more. So can dislike be turned into liking for vegetables? Can food preferences be changed? The science says an overwhelming YES!

In scientific experiments as far back as the 1980s and continuing up to the present day, the incredible effectiveness of 'exposure' has been demonstrated time and time again. What exposure means in this context is repeated tasting – giving a small amount of a particular food on a number of occasions. Done often enough, this changes dislike into liking. It may sound a bit far-fetched, but it is a robust effect seen in animals, children AND adults.

Most of us have experienced the power of exposure without thinking about it. For instance, if you normally take sugar in your tea and then decide to give it up, your first cuppa without it will taste pretty disappointing. Keep at it, though, and after 10 to 15 tries, you will probably find that you like it, and a sugared version no longer tastes right. So it works with all ages – the only thing that differs is the number of times something needs to be tasted before the transformation takes place. As discussed in the previous chapter, infants are particularly receptive to new tastes and may grow to like foods after as few as 3 tries. The reluctant 2- to 5-year-old may need up to 15 tries, as will adolescents and adults.

Some readers may be thinking at this point that their child would never consent to eating a vegetable they don't know or like 15 times. We are here to reassure you that they will, as we have shown in our research. We carried out a series of studies in which children were offered a small piece of a vegetable every day for 15 days and were rewarded with a sticker if they tasted it. We called it the 'Tiny Tastes' game and here's how to do it:

Step 1: Choose a vegetable to try.

Step 2: Choose a regular time of day for the tasting (not mealtimes).

Step 3: Offer a tiny piece (about the size of a 5p piece) and ask the child to taste it.

Step 4: If they comply, give a sticker reward and lots of praise. If they don't taste it, don't give a sticker, but say you will try again the next day.

Step 5: Repeat the next day until the same vegetable has been tasted up to 15 times.

Here are a number of tips to help things along. Firstly, never overwhelm a child by presenting him with large amounts of disliked foods. These tastings need to be of very small amounts that he has helped to cut, if possible. Start by asking him to lick it, maybe place it on his tongue, and always offer a get-out, e.g. 'You can spit it out if you really don't like it.' The sticker rewards should only be given for actual tasting, although spitting out after tasting is allowed. Don't give up until you've managed 15 tastings (only stop before this if the battle has already been won). Research shows that mums typically give up offering something if it has been rejected on 3 to 5 occasions, but you need to persevere for it to work. Quite astonishingly good results have been reported for this type of technique, even with really fussy eaters, and we have produced a pack called 'Tiny Tastes' containing instructions, stickers and monitoring charts which is now available to buy. (See 'Resources and sources of further information' at the end of the book.)

Jo
mum of twins Lilah and Ava (4)

'I think Tiny Tastes works so well because it involves the children and makes it into a game. I can't even remember which vegetable we played it with first because we have done it with so many: tomatoes, sugar snap peas, mushrooms, celery, etc . . . We also used it for new fruits that the twins were reluctant to try. The twins now ask for vegetables and when I cook with mushrooms, I have to chop them up and get them into the pan quickly, otherwise the children will be in the kitchen trying to eat them!'

What else can you do?

As partners in a 4-year Europe-wide project, we have been involved in testing exposure against a variety of other strategies to increase vegetable intake in children from 6 months to 5 years of age. Here are some of them:

- Offering vegetables with a liked dip (e.g. hummus).

- Offering vegetable snacks in interesting shapes (e.g. stars).

- Offering unfamiliar vegetables in the form of a soup.

- Adding spices to improve flavour.

- Involving children in choosing, preparing or growing vegetables.

All of these techniques were moderately successful and all are worth trying, but 'exposure' out-performed all the others. Not only did it increase children's willingness to eat vegetables, but it also made them like them more.

A serving suggestion!

Mums tell us of all sorts of things they've tried, and different techniques work with different children. Sometimes something simple like cooking a vegetable in a different way or serving it raw rather than cooked can change your child's mind about eating it:

Cara

mum of Amelia (3) and Archie (18 months)

'Amelia will often help to get the meals ready which she enjoys, and that's a good opportunity for her to eat raw veg before it goes in the steamer, etc. She'll often eat more veg during meal prep than during the meal itself.'

Like Amelia, many children seem to prefer raw vegetables to cooked ones. The crisp texture of a raw carrot is often more appealing than a soggy, cooked one, so offer chopped-up raw vegetables as snacks or a salad with a meal, and you may find that your child eats a lot more.

The don'ts

Hopefully, we have given you a few new techniques to try, but we can't leave the subject of fruit and vegetables without covering some of the common pitfalls – strategies that we all resort to sometimes, especially when children are refusing all the vegetables on their plate! Beware – these can have unintended consequences:

- **Don't insist that all vegetables are eaten up:** Children who are made to finish something that they really hate may continue to avoid that food for the rest of their lives.[7]

- **Don't offer pudding as a reward for finishing vegetables:** The message that you are giving is that vegetables are so horrible that a reward is needed for anyone managing to eat them. In addition, you are confirming the higher status of sweet foods.

- **Don't hide vegetables in sauces:** Unless every other technique has failed. Children can't get to like something unless they actually taste it.

- **Don't let them know if you don't like vegetables:** If you want your child to eat them, then you should try to eat them too.

---

[7] I am still unable to eat mashed potato or cabbage after the dinner lady, stood over me as I gagged my way through the cold remains of my school dinner in 1966!

TAKE-HOME MESSAGES

- Capitalise on the fact that children are predisposed to like fruit because of its sweetness – just make sure there's lots in the house.

- Always tell children how much you like the foods they are eating.

- Eat plenty of fruit and vegetables yourself and your child will follow suit.

- Give a choice between fruits for pudding and snacks, but not between fruit and some other sweet snack.

- Be persistent – try daily Tiny Tastes and don't give up until you have achieved the magic 15 tastes!

- Try different ways of serving vegetables – sometimes raw is best.

- Offer a liked sauce/dip with new vegetables at first.

- Involve your child in growing, choosing or preparing food.

CHAPTER FIVE

'Picky eaters' and 'plate-clearers'

IN CHAPTER ONE WE TALKED about the differences between children in their attitudes to food. Some are keen eaters who appear to be hungry all the time, enthusiastically finishing all the food on their plate and asking for seconds (food approachers or 'plate-clearers'), while others are picky eaters, rejecting whole groups of foods and appearing to eat virtually nothing while saying that they are full up after a spoonful or two (food avoiders). It's not uncommon to have both types in the same family.

Both of these eating styles can be a significant source of worry to parents. In the case of the plate-clearers, you may worry about current or future weight gain. Fussy or picky children may appear small for their age, and you may be concerned that they are simply not getting enough of anything – calories, vitamins or minerals – to ensure their continued growth.

Penny
mum of Poppy (6) and Stan (2)

'They are very different. Stan eats everything and has a big appetite – he's incredibly active. Poppy is different – she was quite a picky eater, but we've always had a strict rule about trying a little bit of everything. She usually leaves some of her meal – she rarely cleans her plate, unlike Stan. She stops eating when she's had enough.'

In this chapter, we will address the issues arising from having a child at either end of the eating behaviour spectrum, but would stress from the outset that both are very common and, for the vast majority of children, will have no serious consequences. As previously discussed, if you believe that your child is failing to grow adequately or appears significantly overweight, then consult your GP in the first instance.

PICKY EATERS

If you have successfully negotiated the trials and tribulations of weaning, and your rapidly growing offspring is enthusiastically eating a healthy diet high in protein, vegetables and fruit and low in sugary, fatty and processed foods, you may be feeling that you are over the worst, but don't be surprised if things change dramatically during the latter part of the second year. One day, you may sit down at the dinner table and be faced with a total rejection of broccoli, a favourite vegetable 2 days ago; where your 9-month-old baby approached new food with interest and enthusiasm, that same toddler clamps his mouth shut and refuses to have it on his plate. Many parents wonder what they did wrong, whether they have done something to cause their child to start being so choosy, but the answer is usually no. This newly emerging pickiness is a normal and very common behaviour and only a few children pass through their second year without displaying some signs of it.[8]

The term 'picky eater' is used to describe a multitude of different behaviours, but if your child does one or

---

[8] There is a level at which fussy eating ceases to be normal and transient, and an affected child may require more intensive input. Worrying signs might be a loss of weight or faltering growth, or signs of a nutritional deficiency impacting on physical health. Real anxiety around food or rejection of most foods and textures so that the diet consists of only a very small number of possibly age-inappropriate foods would also be a cause for concern. In such rare cases, help should be sought from a GP in the first instance.

more of the following then, by our definition, she would be considered a picky eater:

- Rejects a whole group of foods, e.g. vegetables.
- Has a restricted number of liked foods.
- Doesn't like foods touching on the plate.
- Only likes foods cooked in a certain way.
- Eats slowly.
- Gets full up very quickly.
- Is disinterested in food.

Why are they like this?

As discussed in Chapter 1, these sorts of eating behaviours are inherited from parents to some extent. If you were a very picky eater as a child (or still are, as an adult) then there's a good chance that your child will be too. However, the fact that almost all children display this kind of behaviour at the same sort of age suggests that humans may have evolved to be like this (that it is innate) and, if so, it must have had some useful purpose in our distant past.[9]

---

[9] When we say humans must have evolved this way, we should say that most young omnivorous animals (those that eat a wide variety of different types of foods) are also somewhat wary of unfamiliar foods, supporting the case for this wariness being useful in some way.

For possible explanations for these sorts of questions, we must turn to evolutionary psychologists who seek to explain behaviour in terms of how it would have protected or benefited our cave-dwelling ancestors. In ancient times, food was sourced from the local environment – animals would have been hunted for their meat, and berries, leaves and roots growing in the immediate vicinity would have been gathered by parents and offered to children. Prior to learning to walk at some point in their second year, babies were wholly dependent on their parents to feed them (and, early on, on their mothers only for milk), and could rely on being given foods that were safe to eat. However, once up and running around on their own two feet, children with no fear of unfamiliar foods might pick up and eat potentially toxic or poisonous items with serious if not fatal consequences. Therefore, to be a little wary about foods at this age would have been a useful trait to have. At an earlier stage, most babies will put virtually anything in their mouths, but mums and dads are generally there to keep watch and fish out undesirable objects and substances.

Frustratingly, it always seems to be healthy foods that are rejected by fussy children – rarely do you witness a 2-year-old shying away from an unfamiliar type of biscuit or a different flavour of ice cream. The fact is that study after study has shown that the foods most often rejected by picky children are, in typical order of dislike: vegetables, fruit and then protein foods (meat and fish). No effect of fussiness has been seen on intake of starchy, fatty, sugary or dairy foods.

This makes perfect sense if you consider that plant and protein foods pose the most significant risk of poisoning to young children. Toxins are present in many plants (vegetables and fruits), while animal foods (meat, fish and eggs) are primary sources of bacteria, causing food poisoning. However, the food supply has never been safer than in the present day and this tendency towards food refusal may now be an adaptation that humans would be better off without. Unfortunately, evolution is a very slow process and the pre-disposition for 2-year-olds to reject foods is unlikely to disappear any time soon.

Mealtimes with a fussy eater

Having a picky eater in the family can be extremely stressful, turning mealtimes into a battle of wills and parents into anxious wrecks. Feeding a child is an emotive business – knowing that your child has had a good, wholesome meal feels really good, whereas a fraught mealtime can be frustrating and worrying.

Cara
mum of Amelia (3) and Archie (18 months)

'A meal with Amelia usually starts with "I don't like [insert dinner]"! Unless it's fish fingers! I usually reassure her that she enjoyed it last time and encourage her to sit nicely and show her little brother how to eat like a big girl. She'll eat a bit and then ask for help (for me to feed her) or to "make a deal" because she doesn't want any more. Recently I've tried to use more distraction – talk to her about something other than food, reflect on the day, plan what we'll do later, and she'll often get on and eat a bit more. More often than not I feed her the final few mouthfuls and she usually leaves about 20 per cent of what was on her plate. It gets quite wearing, having the same conversations every mealtime, always having to encourage, and I usually end up feeding her as I get fed up of how slowly she's eating! But I'm hoping she will grow out of it and I try my best not to lose my patience, though sometimes she does get told to stop moaning and eat her tea, or she'll be very bored because she's having to sit at the table for such a long time!'

Will she grow out of it?

Children are at their most picky between the ages of 2 and 5 years. In most, it will decline after this and they will gradually expand their dietary repertoire over later childhood, adolescence and adulthood. However, some will remain fussy about food for much longer than this, especially those with a genetic predisposition to be so. Apart from being difficult for parents to deal with, a lack of dietary variety and low intake of fruit and vegetables is bad news for health, so it really is worth trying to nip the problem in the bud.

What you can do to help

The important thing to remember is that the two characteristics that most strongly predict a child's liking for, and willingness to eat, something are its sweetness and the extent to which it looks (and then tastes) familiar.

Role models

Documenters of animal eating behaviour have observed that young monkeys, birds and many other species will not eat an unfamiliar-looking food until they have observed an older animal eating it and experiencing no adverse consequences (illness or death!). Only then will they try it themselves – this is known as 'learned safety', and baby humans have to learn it, too.

So, how can you make the foods you want your child to eat seem safe and familiar? Firstly, we have said this before but never underestimate the importance of role models, especially parents. Your child looks up to you, wants to be like you, and knows that you can show her which foods are good tasting, nutritious and, crucially, safe. This means you have to eat vegetables and other healthy foods with enthusiasm in front of her – tell her that it tastes great and that you love it!

The presence of enthusiastic friends is also highly influential, as Georgina illustrates here:

Georgina
mum of Emily (4)

'Emily was going through this funny phase where she wouldn't eat broccoli when she always used to. When her playmate from nursery was over for tea one evening I bought some pizza bases and sauce and put sweetcorn, mushrooms,

cherry tomatoes, peppers, broccoli and grated cheese in different bowls and we played Mr and Mrs Pizza Face. We all made a different pizza face using the vegetables – broccoli as the hair, mushroom as the nose, cherry tomatoes as the eyes and so on. We then ate a bit of each of the pizzas. Emily ate a bit of everything – I couldn't believe it! – without flinching. It was either because Jo her friend was there or the pizza-face game – I don't know!'

Exposure: increasing familiarity with daily tasting

Chapter 4 has a full description of the most effective means of increasing liking and intake of fruit and (especially) vegetables – repeated taste exposure, or 'Tiny Tastes' as we have named it. The technique can be successfully used for any food that is a problem.

Don't lose control

It's tempting with picky eaters to just give them the few foods that they like and to give up on trying anything new: many parents end up cooking two different dishes in order to ensure that their fussy toddler eats something at mealtimes, but with gentle encouragement and lots of praise you'll get there in the end.

Rest assured, most children will grow out of this picky stage eventually, but there are things you can do to speed up the process:

Top tips for feeding picky eaters

- Be a role model – eat the foods that you are trying to get your child to eat.

- Expose your child to a variety of different foods – familiarity leads to liking.

- Try the 'Tiny Tastes' technique with disliked foods.

- Gently encourage your child to try at least some of the food and praise them when they have tasted it.

- Involve your child in food preparation.

Beware of supplements for fussy eaters!

Recently, nutritional powdered milkshakes have appeared on the shelves that are mixed with water and come in different flavours, such as vanilla, strawberry or chocolate. They deliver over 220 calories per serving, and 2 servings a day are recommended for under 5s (3 for over 5s). That is a lot of calories and a lot of sugar – nearly 34 grams in 2 servings, which is nearly 8 teaspoons of sugar – for something that is to be used 'alongside or between meals'.

Ingredients generally include:

Hydrolysed corn starch, sugar, milk proteins, soy oil, high oleic sunflower oil, medium chain triglycerides from palm kernel oil, soy protein isolate, fructooligosaccharides powder, potassium citrate, flavouring, magnesium phosphate, potassium chloride, sodium chloride, calcium phosphate, potassium phosphate, docosahexaenoic acid (DHA) (soy), choline chloride, calcium carbonate, vitamin C, arachidonic acid (AA) (soy), taurine, m-inositol, ferrous sulphate, carnitine tartrate, Lactobacillus acidophilus, antioxidant: E306, vitamin E, zinc sulphate, calcium pantothenate, niacin, Bifidobacterium lactis, manganese sulphate, vitamin B6, vitamin B1, vitamin B2, vitamin A, copper sulphate, folic acid, potassium iodide, chromium chloride, sodium selenite, vitamin K, sodium molybdate, biotin, vitamin D3, vitamin B12.

Make no mistake, these milkshakes will fill your child up and deliver lots of vitamins. The trouble is that having drunk a glass of this sweet milkshake, no child is going to have any appetite for good, healthy, *real* food. In addition, if offered 'alongside' meals 2 or 3 times a day, there is a real risk of excess weight gain. We have spoken out against this type of product, as have experts in feeding disorders in the USA[10], and would strongly advise trying our behavioural approaches on your fussy eater rather than these quick-fix food substitutes.

Now we will look at the other end of the spectrum – the avid eaters or 'plate-clearers'.

PLATE-CLEARERS

We would define a plate-clearer as a child who is enthusiastic about food and displays these sorts of behaviours:

- Eats quickly.

- Always seems hungry.

- Never seems to be full.

- Finishes everything on his plate and asks for more (or pinches food off other children's plates!).

- Looks forward to mealtimes.

---

[10] www.telegraph.co.uk/foodanddrink/11000235/The-Kitchen-Thinker-can-a-calorific-milkshake-really-help-fussy-eaters.html

- Wants snacks soon after mealtimes.

Plate-clearers are often, but not always, good eaters from birth, avidly devouring milk and wanting frequent feeds. This sounds like the opposite of picky eating, but like their picky counterparts, these children may also dislike fruit and vegetables so some of the techniques previously discussed may come in handy.

Whilst it is rewarding to have a child who appreciates your culinary efforts, many parents will be concerned about the potential for excess weight gain and accompanying health and social issues.

Maggie
mum of Gemma (7) and Tom (5)

'My children are really different eaters. Tom isn't interested in food, while Gemma, well, we have to keep her out of the fridge. We put a lock on it at one point because she would just help herself to string-cheese snacks. She came home from school the other day saying someone had called her fat. We are quite strict with ensuring they eat healthy foods, but with Gemma she is always hungry.'

Weight issues

Childhood overweight and obesity has increased dramatically in recent years and therefore parents are entirely right to be concerned. However, recent research indicates that parents are very poor at identifying when their own child is overweight and may be reluctant to do anything about it for fear of 'making it an issue' or of increasing the likelihood of their child developing an eating disorder. In parents' defence, it is extremely difficult to judge whether a child under 5 years of age is overweight, but the earlier a weight problem is identified, the greater is the chance that it can be overcome. Generally speaking, without intervention, an overweight child will become an overweight adolescent and then an overweight adult, as the longer excess weight stays on, the harder it is to lose.

Before taking any action you need to establish whether or not your child is actually overweight. In the UK, children are weighed and measured at the start of formal schooling and feedback is given to parents as to their child's weight status. Prior to that, an indication of a potential problem might be that your child is wearing clothes in a size for a much older child, or if the clothes that fit in height are much too small in the waist. There are websites[11] where you can find a calculator to assess your child's BMI (body mass index – the accepted medical measure of weight status), or see your GP or practice nurse.

If your child is identified as being overweight or obese then the best thing you can do is to look at the family diet and level of activity and try to make sure that everyone in the family is eating the types of food that are high in nutritional value and low in salt and sugar. It sounds obvious, but try not to single out your child to be fed differently – the whole family will benefit from eating healthily and getting plenty of exercise. There is little point in talking to very young children about their weight – better to simply talk about how good it feels to be healthy and active. Avoid being critical of your own or anyone else's weight and NEVER describe your child as being 'chubby', or similar.

---

[11] www.weightconcern.org.uk has a BMI calculator and lots of advice for tackling excess weight gain in children.

Cara

mum of Amelia (3) and Archie (18 months)

'Amelia is about average weight, and I think and we feel like she has a good variety of food, with occasional treats. Archie is bigger, nearer to the 90th percentile, but I control his portions and he has healthy food and is slimming down now that he is walking. I was concerned when he was younger that he was eating too much and adjusted how I fed him a bit, i.e. only filled the spoon again when he opened his mouth for it, rather than having the next one ready.'

Regardless of weight status, some children are just hungrier than others, and the way you respond to an avid appetite is important. Simply forbidding sweets and snacks may backfire by making them even more desirable to your child – the 'forbidden fruit' effect.

One of the most useful skills that these children can learn is what has been termed 'self-regulation'. In plain English, this means the ability to recognise when you are full and when you are hungry, and to respond appropriately to both. What follows is guidance in how to help your child to have a healthy relationship with food: eating when they are hungry and, most importantly, knowing when to stop.

Controlling and restricting

In the plentiful food environment of the twenty-first century, you are going to have to exert some control over what your child eats, restricting their access to the vast array of junk foods on offer. However, research has emerged to suggest that the *way* in which parents control their children's food intake has a profound influence on their eating behaviour – and not always a good one.

In a neat experiment in a US day-care centre, children were given unlimited access to one type of cookie at snack time; on the same table, in full view, was a clear storage jar containing a different type of cookie – one that the children liked just as much. For a few minutes in the middle of snack time, the lid of the storage jar was opened and children were allowed to consume these other cookies before the lid was then replaced. What the researchers found was that after this experience, the children said that they preferred the cookies that they had been partially prevented from eating. By being restricted, those cookies had become more desirable.

Although this was only a one-off experiment, it is easy to see that if children know that there is something that they're not allowed to have, they actually want it more, not less. These findings have led scientists to conclude that overt and very strict restriction of unhealthy foods is counter-productive. Therefore, when dealing with your child's enthusiasm for snacks, try to avoid the kind of response described below:

Josie
mum of Alfie (6)

'I'm actually going to put a lock on one of my cupboards and put crisps and stuff like that in it because my son just doesn't know when to stop and I need to sometimes address that.'

By responding like this, Josie is 'over-controlling' the situation, which is likely to lead Alfie to want the things that he is forbidden from having even more. Research studies support this view and suggest that children who have been restricted may eat more when they are given the opportunity, even if they are not hungry.

Techniques now emerging from the scientific research seem promising. Much more effective than very strict restriction appears to be a sort of 'covert' control involving the removal of temptation – simply avoiding bringing 'problem' foods into the house. After all, if it's not there, they can't have it (and nor will you need to lock it away!). Perhaps not surprisingly, a number of research studies have shown that children have a better diet, eating more fruit and vegetables and fewer unhealthy foods in homes where unhealthy foods are not available.

Using food to reward, entertain or comfort

While we have strongly promoted the use of stickers to reward good healthy eating, food rewards are a real no-no. The classic: 'Eat your peas and you can have some ice cream' strategy simply teaches children that peas are horrible and ice cream is special. Studies show that after experiencing this sort of bargaining over food, children like peas less, and ice cream more, than they did before. Avoiding this is not always easy, but this mum has developed a way of focusing on the positive benefits of the healthiest parts of the meal.

Cara
mum of Amelia (3) and Archie (18 months)

'I try to avoid rewarding food with food but it's extremely difficult to say why Amelia can't eat her pudding until she's eaten more of her meal without saying, "You need to finish your pasta before you have a yoghurt." Now she's a bit older I try to talk to her about how foods help us to grow, strengthen our muscles, give us energy, etc. So I will say it's important to eat your meal (pasta/shepherds pie, etc.) so you have lots of energy to run around and play, and fruit and vegetables will help you to grow strong and healthy, and ice cream is yummy too, but it's not so good at helping us grow or run fast so you need to eat the other things too.'

It's tempting to give sweets or a packet of crisps to a bored and grumpy child while you are out shopping, or to provide a distraction from the pain of a grazed knee, but the result is likely to be a habit of eating when bored or sad, which may persist into adulthood and be very difficult to break. Many adults who struggle with their weight report that they comfort-eat, so try to offer hugs for comfort and toys or games to entertain instead of food.

Portion sizes

The amount that you put on your child's plate will dictate how much they eat. In an intriguing experiment carried out in the USA, 3- and 5-year-old children were given age-appropriate portion sizes of macaroni cheese on one occasion and double portions on another day. Interestingly, the 3-year-olds ate roughly the same amount regardless of how much was on their plate, but the 5-year-olds ate significantly more when given a larger serving. The authors concluded that 3-year-olds are able to stop eating when they are full even if there is food left on their plate, whereas 5-year-olds will go on eating if food is available. The reason why older children appear to lose the ability to recognise when they are full is uncertain, but what is clear is that you can manipulate how much they eat by offering smaller portions at first. Don't forget, children's tummies are much smaller than grown-ups' – adult portions are too big for under-5s. If they are genuinely still hungry after a first helping then they can be given seconds, but it's worth waiting a short while to allow them to experience their feeling of fullness. Talk to them about what it feels like to be hungry or full. This will help them to pay more attention to these feelings and less to the mere presence of food.

Eating speed

In a similar vein, teaching children to eat more slowly – perhaps putting the knife and fork down between mouthfuls – will give the food time to reach their stomachs and make it easier for them to recognise when they get full up.

Family mealtimes

Although it isn't always easy to arrange, eating together as a family provides a great learning opportunity for children and may improve the diet of the parents as well, as Cara describes:

Cara

mum of Amelia (3) and Archie (18 months)

'The days I don't work we try to eat as a family and Tom and I have to modify what we eat a little to suit the children, i.e. not much salt/spices. The children enjoy it when we all sit together. The challenge is finding the time to make a meal while trying to play with the children. Archie is too young to really play with Amelia so a lot of time is spent trying to entertain them on separate tasks, and cooking at the same time can be hard work! Where possible I do most of the cooking/preparation when they have their afternoon nap, to try and limit how much I have to do at teatime.'

Even if you only manage to have a family mealtime once a week, it's worth doing. Your child can help you prepare the meal, you can model healthy eating behaviour and talk about how good the food tastes, and you can monitor the amount your child is eating. Serve the same food (in appropriate portion sizes) to everyone, and turn off the TV so that everyone can pay attention to what they are eating.

Avoid pressurising a child to eat more than they want to – this is another way in which we may override a child's feelings of fullness, as well as making mealtimes stressful. Within reason, allow her to decide *how much* she eats while you decide *what* she eats. Don't put more on her plate if she says she's not hungry and don't spoon in the last two mouthfuls, no matter how tempting it is to hurry the meal along.

Snacking

If your child has a big appetite you may feel that you should try to limit their snacking, but very young children can rarely manage with only 3 meals a day. Don't forget that snacks are a great opportunity to get more fruit or vegetables down your children – a banana sandwich, or carrot sticks and hummus are great choices. Try to monitor their intake – in other words, limit and keep track of the unhealthy foods they consume, but a biscuit or some crisps every now and then is fine.

Top tips for feeding plate-clearers

- Avoid the 'forbidden fruit' effect – only bring the foods you want your child to eat into the house.

- Use stickers rather than food to reward your child for eating well.

- Avoid giving food to comfort or entertain.

- Be aware of portion sizes – children will eat more if you give them more.

- Snack time is a great way to try out new fruit and vegetables.

Just to sum up . . . the tips below should help you to understand and deal with the big and little eaters, but do try to maintain a sense of humour. Feeding children can be stressful, but staying calm is vital and will stop mealtimes becoming something everyone dreads and no one enjoys.

TAKE-HOME MESSAGES

- A period of fussy eating and rejection of unfamiliar foods is very common in the toddler years and is a normal stage of development.

- The foods that are most often refused are vegetables, fruits and meat or fish.

- Act as a role model by eating healthily and being enthusiastic about the taste.

- Repeated exposure to tiny tastes of foods outside mealtimes and with a sticker reward if necessary, can alter preferences.

- Give lots of praise for good eating.

- Help your child to be aware of the feelings of hunger and fullness. Never use food as a reward or to entertain or comfort.

- Keep lots of healthy foods in the house and keep the unhealthy ones out!

- Don't make your child finish everything on their plate.

- Turn off the TV at mealtimes.

- Eat together as a family whenever you can.

- Parents should decide what to eat, and allow children to decide how much.

CHAPTER SIX

Friends, relatives and childcare: a force for good or evil?

WHILE YOU ARE THE sole person in charge of your child's food intake, you may be able to keep them from even knowing that junk and processed foods exist. However, as soon as a child spends time away from home with friends and relatives, or in childcare, there's a danger that all the hard work that you put in to engender healthy eating habits will be undone. Grandparents may give too many sweet treats, other children's parents may be less concerned about dietary quality than you are, and nursery schools may give sweet rewards for good behaviour. On the plus side, children will often try things away from home that they would point-blank refuse at home and the power of peer pressure should never be underestimated – sharing a meal with a best friend who eats all their vegetables can encourage fussier children to try a taste themselves. This chapter will address the positive and negative impact of outsiders on your child's food preferences and eating behaviour, and show how you can turn significant others into a force for good.

CHILDCARE – INFORMAL AND FORMAL[12]

Let's start with some facts and figures:

- Roughly 80 per cent of 3–6 year olds and 25 per cent of children aged less than 3 years are in some form of childcare in OECD[13] countries, mostly in order to allow parents to return to work.

- 76 per cent of parents of young children work part-time or full-time and the majority use at least some informal care, the overwhelming majority of which is provided by grandparents.

- Between 4 and 7 million grandparents provide childcare, 20 per cent for more than 10 hours a week.

- This saves parents about £7 billion – no small amount!

The popularity of grandparental care is clear and most parents believe that it offers the next best thing to full-time parental care, especially with regard to the emotional well-being of the child. For parents working atypical or variable hours, there may be

---

[12] By formal, we mean in a nursery or other childcare centre, with a registered childminder, nanny or au pair. Informal care is that provided by relatives or friends or unregistered childminders.

[13] Organisation for Economic Co-operation and Development.

no alternative care available and, of course, formal childcare costs may be out of reach for many families.

Informal care

Although many of the issues discussed will apply to other informal carers, we will focus in this section on the impact of care by grandparents, as they form the largest proportion of informal caregivers.

Typically, grandparents are an overwhelming force for good in a child's life. It has been said that children cared for by grandparents have larger vocabularies and are less likely to have behaviour problems, although some research suggests that they may be less school-ready than those cared for solely by mothers or in formal care. There is far less research into their impact on children's eating habits, although there has been quite a lot of interest in whether grandparental care has an effect on children's body weight. In a number of studies conducted in the US, Canada and UK, being cared for by a grandparent is associated with a higher risk of overweight and obesity, as is care by other members of the family or by neighbours, although two studies from Japan found no such association. It's hard to come to a conclusion on this issue, as differences between the studies may well be due to cultural differences.

What might grandparents be doing wrong?

Online forums periodically buzz with livid mums complaining about how their parents and in-laws feed their children fizzy drinks, chocolates and sweets, undermining all their attempts to instil healthy eating habits. It seems to be a very common problem.

Alice
mum of Nick (16 months)

'When they do have him they let him have far more sweet things than I would ideally like and they also let him watch more TV – in the 2 weeks that we stayed with them so they could help out with childcare whilst Nick's childminder was away, he learnt to say the name of his favourite channel!!! It's funny because when I was little we were never allowed cakes, biscuits or sweets and we certainly never ate in front of the telly. When I said this to my mum, she said that it was what you are supposed do as a grandparent – spoil your grandchildren and give them treats.'

Alice's point is an interesting one. The way we feed our children is usually very similar to the way we were fed by our parents, but when faced with their darling grandchildren, they abandon all the rules we had to abide by and spoil them rotten!

Here's one grandfather's side of the story . . .

Sam
grandfather of Jessica (5)

'We give Jessica treats – let her have sausage and chips when we're out . . . we probably feed her bad foods really, and just hope she eats all right when she's at home. When we look after her during the week we make food at home. We give her novelty cheeses because she likes that but we give her tomatoes and cucumber with it too. We give her lots of fruits but she doesn't like blueberries and pears and we don't know where that comes from. What I think is that as long as she eats well at home we can give her treats when we're out.'

So, apart from giving too many sweets, what are the other reasons why children might gain weight in their grandparents' care?

Activity

Some reasons that spring to mind are to do with exercise. Some grandparents may not be as fit as they were and may not be agile or mobile enough to offer much in the way of physical activity. This may be why they resort to the TV as entertainment more often than going to the park. Another reason may be that parents' knowledge about nutrition is far greater now than it was when grandparents were bringing up their own children. Grandparents may not be so aware of the need to restrict or control your child's intake of certain foods. Quite the reverse; the belief in the necessity of finishing all the food on your plate was widely held in years gone by and was borne of the relative scarcity of food experienced by the previous post-war generation.

Feeding practices

Another reason may be that the feeding techniques that they use are not the most effective at getting children to eat healthily. We know that parental feeding practices have a profound effect on children's food preferences, eating habits, attitudes to food and weight (see Chapter 5 for a detailed description of effective and ineffective strategies). It's likely that the strategies that grandparents use when feeding their grandchildren are also highly influential on a child's growing relationship with food.

Kate
mum of Ben (18 months)

'Probably the most infuriating thing my mother-in-law does is feed him with a spoon, when he doesn't need this (she likes him to be a baby, and need her, whereas I like to see him progressing through the development stages and being independent!). The reason it winds me up is that he doesn't get the chance to realise when he's full and stop. Sometimes I can see he doesn't want to eat any more and she's still trying to squash it into his mouth. Makes me think of a foie gras goose!'

On the other hand, some grandparents may actually provide healthier meal foods, simply because they may have more time than busy working parents:

Kate
mum of Ben (18 months)

'My mum nearly always cooks from scratch and when she's feeding Ben, would never resort to a short cut, unlike me. If I'm pushed for time I will give Ben a fresh ready-meal but my mum would never do this, as she thinks it's full of junk, is a waste of money, and she'd prefer to make it herself so she knows what's in it. Although she would never dream of using a ready-made meal, she admits it's different for me as 3 or 4 days a week I only get home at dinner time, so need to get food on the table quickly, and only have an hour with Ben before bedtime, so don't want to spend 15 minutes standing at the hob.'

The science

There is a real scarcity of research into the feeding practices of formal and informal caregivers in general, and grandparents in particular. One exception is a study of Chinese 3-generation families (in which grandparents live with their children), which found that grandparents frequently use food to express love and care, and have a tendency to over-feed by giving over-large portions at mealtimes. Of course, the typical family set-up in Western societies is very different to that in China, where grandparents frequently live with their children and grandchildren and therefore have considerably more involvement and influence on child feeding.

Nevertheless, recent research from the UK into the feeding practices of parents and grandparents has provided some insight into what goes on when Granny is in charge of mealtimes, and the news is not all bad! Some grandparents do see their role as providing even better, healthier food than the child might be getting at home.

In one study, grandparents reported trying to keep plenty of healthy foods in the house and less unhealthy cakes, ice cream and sweets than parents, and the more time they spent looking after their grandchildren, the more common this was. However, it emerged that their feeding practices were not always the best for helping children to develop a healthy relationship with food. For example, grandparents are very keen on offering food as a reward or as comfort – both of which can have unintended consequences. This is covered in more detail in Chapter 5, but you don't have to have a PhD in psychology to work out that if children are given sweets or cakes when they are upset, they will rapidly start to see food as something to turn to when they feel sad or lonely – to become emotional eaters, in other words. These sorts of associations are hard to break and it would be best to gently ask Granny to find other sources of reward or comfort, like stickers, or cuddles or being read a story.

Another thing that grandparents do that drives mums mad is to give too much control to their grandchildren. Decisions over what, where and how much to eat, how much television is allowed, when bedtime is, and sundry other choices may be given to children with predictable results when they get back to you again – rebellion! Telling a very young child that what happens at Granny's house doesn't happen at home doesn't always do the trick.

As an aside, your mum or dad may not tell you, but some of them don't think too highly of the way you are managing things, as this grandfather told us:

Mark
grandfather of Will (4) and Sophie (8 months)

'We don't look after the grandchildren very often, but we were just in France for a week with them. What I see is that my children are feeding their children too much – my 4-year-old grandson got 2 and half scrambled eggs for breakfast. And there's so much waste. Then my daughter is weaning her daughter by getting her to feed herself and pick up foods. Most of it ends up on the floor (which our dog loves)!

What can you do?

Lots of tact on both sides is probably the way forward, but the extent to which feeding issues are a real problem depends largely on how much time children remain in grandparents' care. The occasional day of junk food and TV won't do too much harm and for the sake of peace you may be best advised to ignore it, but if you have to rely on a spoiling grandparent for regular childcare, it's a bit trickier. If you are not paying for their time, it will be more difficult to lay down the law, but in the long run grandparents want the best for their grandchildren and a calm conversation about how you would like them to treat your child and why will go a long way. Suggest that instead of sweet treats or toys, your child could have a story read to them or play a special game as a reward or for comfort. Don't be too disappointed if your requests are ignored. Some grandparents really do think it's their right to spoil their grandchildren:

Penny
mum of Poppy (6) and Stan (2)

'When the children go to stay with my in-laws they have tea (the children have milk) and biscuits in bed in the morning before getting up and going downstairs for breakfast. This is something that they used to do with my husband and his brother at the weekends when they were little. I have always said that I would rather that they didn't but there are some battles not worth fighting. The rest of the time they feed them healthy things and encourage them to eat fruit and vegetables.'

Grandparents won't be around forever and the benefits of the unique relationship they have with your child will almost always outweigh the negative effect of the occasional bag of chocolate buttons.

Formal childcare

Formal care, in the form of kindergarten, nursery school, or with a registered childminder has not been associated with higher child-weight in most studies, although some have found that anything other than sole maternal care confers a slightly greater risk of overweight. Of course, this is manna from heaven to the *Daily Mail* columnists who are always happy to feature findings that support the view that a woman's place is in the home!

Published in March 2014 and effective from September 2014, the Statutory Framework for the Early Years Foundation Stage (children aged 0–5 years) states that:

> *'Where children are provided with meals, snacks and drinks, they must be healthy, balanced and nutritious. Before a child is admitted to the setting, the provider must also obtain information about*

any special dietary requirements, preferences and food allergies that the child has, and any special health requirements. Fresh drinking water must be available and accessible at all times. Providers must record and act on information from parents and carers about a child's dietary needs.'

They must also inform you of the food and drink that they make available to your child. However, there is no definition of 'healthy, balanced and nutritious' and there are currently no legally binding or enforceable guidelines, although the School Food Trust has produced a practical guide for childcare providers.[14] What is allowed outside meals in schools varies tremendously and can be unhelpful for parents wanting to limit sugary food consumption.

---

[14] www.childrensfoodtrust.org.uk/pre-school/resources/guidelines

Penny
mother of Poppy (6) and Stan (2)

'The school allows the children to bring in sweets for their class if it's their birthday which I don't really agree with, but you have to do it if all the other children do. Also every Friday there is a cake sale so they always come home with some cake. They have really strict rules about packed lunches though – no sweets and so on. It's all a bit contradictory.'

However, there is much good practice in early-years childcare these days and, anecdotally, parents often report that their child has eaten things at nursery that they would point-blank refuse at home. The sorts of strategies that have been found to be especially effective are:

- Offering fruit and vegetables at snack time rather than biscuits and cake.

- Staff sitting with children and encouraging them to try new things.

- Involving children in setting tables and preparing and serving food.

- Playing games in which children try to identify healthy and unhealthy foods.

Recent research conducted in Welsh nursery schools found that childcare practitioners were mostly using highly effective child-feeding strategies such as modelling and gentle encouragement, while permitting children some autonomy over how much they ate. A further study of Liverpool day-care settings found a less rosy picture, with staff in need of better training and support, but nevertheless reported that nurseries were '. . . genuinely interested in providing appropriate healthy food for under-5s'. A study in the USA showed how influential childcare practitioners can be on children's eating, reporting that gentle encouragement from staff to eat more was highly effective in getting children to eat more fruit and vegetables. This is consistent with previous research looking at the impact of teachers sitting with children at mealtimes and making positive remarks about the food provided. Just saying: 'Yum! I love mangoes,' got a significant number of reluctant eaters to try it in one study.

Of course, the other influential factor in childcare

settings is other children and all that they bring to the party. First and foremost, your child's peers are models for all sorts of behaviours, including eating. Children want to do what their friends do and a large body of research shows that watching friends eating and enjoying something will greatly increase the chances of them doing likewise. Which brings us to the final section in this chapter – the impact of your child's social life.

THE PERILS AND BENEFITS OF A SOCIAL LIFE

Once your child starts nursery, if not before, friendships with other children will start to be established. That will mean meals in other people's houses, and other people's children eating at your house with all sorts of implications, good and bad. Firstly, the bad news: if your child's friends normally sit down to processed turkey shapes and potato shapes, then your child is on the road to discovering a whole world of 'children's foods' that you may have managed to keep secret until now. In all likelihood your child will love these and come home asking if you can get them when you next go shopping. SAY NO! DO NOT WAVER! Once you have given in, all is lost! Calmly explain that different people eat different foods and that those aren't foods that your family eats, but that it's OK if he eats them when he is out to tea. When that child comes to a meal with your child, don't make concessions – serve what you would normally serve. You may be doing the child's mum a big favour by introducing him to some new foods. Conversely, you could get lucky if your child is a fussy eater and his friend is a real plate-clearer: some of the friend's enthusiasm for food will almost certainly rub off on your child.

Parties are another potentially rich source of palatable junk food. You might get lucky and have a child like Caitlin's son:

Caitlin
mum of Tim (10), Lily (8) and George (4)

'When George goes . . . to others' birthday parties, there are often chicken nuggets (my nemesis), lollipops and doughnuts. Apart from sweets, we don't stop him having such treats at birthday parties, as we don't feel that's fair. But, as we've discovered, he makes "good choices" – parents have told us he has declined cake and asked instead for watermelon, and always chooses water.'

. . . but it's unlikely! Again, explain that party food is not for every day and resign yourself to the fact that it's the price you pay for having a sociable child.

A word of warning . . . there are children who get extremely anxious when eating meals at someone else's house or anywhere away from home. She won't thank me for using her as an example, but my eldest daughter used to cry every day at school when faced with her school lunch because she didn't recognise the food on offer and didn't want to try it. At the same time, she knew that she *should* eat because everyone else was eating and it was expected of her. In the end, we had to give in and provide her with a packed lunch every day instead. What you really don't want to do is force the issue with a child like her, as there is a danger of engendering some very negative feelings around food that may persist.

HOLIDAYS WITH OTHER FAMILIES

This always sounds like a great idea – providing company for you and your children. You imagine reciprocal babysitting and children happily playing together, allowing you to relax and let someone else build the sandcastle for a change. Unfortunately, unless you know the other family very well and have done some groundwork beforehand, things can be pretty stressful, especially with regard to snacks and mealtimes. Even your closest friends or relatives, with whom you believe you share the same values and beliefs, may turn a blind eye to things that you wouldn't dream of allowing.

It is a really good idea to have a chat beforehand to try to agree some rules about what is and isn't allowed in the way of treats and general eating behaviour while you are away. You may need to compromise a little for the sake of a peaceful life and an ongoing friendship. If the other family plans to abandon any pretence of healthy eating for the duration of the holiday, you may want to try to negotiate a sort of one-day-on, one-day-off arrangement, but if it looks as though it's going to be a deal-breaker, consider backing down. It's only a week (or a fortnight) and there's very little real damage going to be done. Again, try to explain to your child that there will be a temporary departure from normal food rules, but that they will be reinstated when the holiday is over.

We've been a bit pessimistic here – an alternative scenario is that the other children are paragons of gastronomic virtue and will be great role models for your child, enthusiastically putting away piles of green vegetables at mealtimes. If that were the case, a few too many ice creams would be a small price to pay for your child's newfound love of spinach!

TAKE-HOME MESSAGES

- Children will often try a new food away from home that they regularly refuse at home – capitalise on this and draft in help from grandparents and friends to introduce problem foods like vegetables when your child is with them.

- Children will imitate the eating behaviour of anyone they admire – that means you, but also relatives, teachers, friends and childcare workers.

- Grandparents have a tendency to spoil their grandchildren with treats and privileges not allowed at home. Indulge this to some extent, but try to agree some boundaries.

- A chicken nugget or potato waffle now and then won't undo all the good work you've done – relax!

CHAPTER SEVEN

The enemy within:
screen time

MOST CHILDREN LOVE WATCHING television and it can be
a useful tool to educate, reward, entertain or soothe.
However, watching too much TV can have a negative
impact upon children's health, diet, weight and activity
levels. Recommendations state that children under
the age of 2 years shouldn't watch TV at all, while
children over 2 should watch no more than 2 hours
a day. Yet, many children watch far more than this
and are increasingly using other types of screen media,
such as online games and mobile apps, exposing them
to advertisements for all sorts of products including
sweet, salty and fatty foods and sweetened drinks.

It has been estimated that children in the USA watch
between 23,000 and 40,000 television ads a year, with
similar levels documented in Europe and Australia.[15]
Advertised foods are rarely healthy and excess

---

[15] E. Neuborne, 'For Kids on the Web, It's an Ad, Ad, Ad, Ad
World', Business Week 3475 (13 August 2001), 108–109

exposure to these ads can undermine your attempts to feed your child a balanced diet. Manufacturers aggressively market their most unhealthy products to children, some as young as 2 years old. One study from Yale University showed that cereals advertised to children contained 57 per cent more sugar, 52 per cent less fibre, and 50 per cent more salt compared with adult-targeted cereals.

This chapter describes the findings of research into the impact of TV viewing and other screen media on children's activity levels, food intake and food requests.

THE EFFECT OF TV WATCHING

Mums have told us how useful TV is to them:

Jane
mum of Ella (2)

'We have just managed to get Ella to watch children's TV between 6.30 and 7 which really calms her down and makes it easier for me to put her PJs on and give her her milk. This makes her sleep better because she's wound down and calm.'

Alice
mum of Nick (16 months)

'Nick watches about half an hour of TV in the mornings sometimes, just so that I can get on with getting ready to go to work. He only ever watches children's TV or things we have recorded. We don't let him watch much at all, unless he's not well and too tired to play. Then it comes in handy.'

Annie
mum of Jake (18 months)

'Jake has just got into watching animated feature films which is great. It gives us 15 minutes of peace while we're getting breakfast ready, sorting chores and things. Before, Jake would be hanging off of our legs (often wailing) while we were trying to get his milk ready.'

It's worth knowing that children who watch a lot of TV seem to have worse diets than those who watch less or no TV. Evidence is also emerging of a link between screen time and weight gain. There are a number of reasons that have been suggested to explain this link. Firstly and most obviously, children who are watching the TV are sitting down instead of running about getting some exercise. Secondly, children who eat their meals in front of the TV tend to eat more, perhaps because it distracts them from paying attention to how full they are. Finally, being exposed to lots of advertisements for unhealthy foods makes children want these products, and to pester you to buy them.

Let's look at these effects in more detail:

Children are sedentary when watching TV

Being sedentary for long periods is bad for everyone's health. Over recent years, the prevalence of overweight and obesity in children has increased dramatically, while fitness has decreased. Data from the US reports that 2- to 5-year-old children spend more than 32 hours a week on average in front of a TV screen – that's 4.5 hours a day![16] – while data

---

[16] www.nielsen.com/us/en/insights/news/2009/tv-viewing-among-kids-at-an-eight-year-high.html

from the UK shows that over 70 per cent of children do not meet recommendations for under-5s, which are to be active for 3 hours every day.

It's important to encourage physical activity from birth. Babies who cannot yet crawl can still be encouraged to reach and grasp, pull and push and move their legs and arms. Once they are crawling, children should be encouraged to move as much as possible within a safe environment. The first 2 years of life are critical for brain development, and TV and other screen media can get in the way of children exploring, interacting and playing with others, which helps them to learn and to develop socially and physically.

Once children can walk, they should be active for at least 3 hours a day and this can take many forms: playing games (e.g. hide and seek), ball games, fast walking, cycling, dancing, swimming, climbing, skipping, rolling, jumping and so on.

Why is activity important?

Physical activity is key for:

• Promoting well-being and reducing anxiety and depression.

- Boosting self-esteem.
- Contributing to maintaining a healthy weight.
- Improving children's cognitive development (e.g. language, information processing, perception and other aspects of brain development).
- Improving physical health and preventing diseases such as heart disease and diabetes in later life.
- Strengthening the immune system.
- Aiding sleep.

Children eat more when watching TV

A wealth of research has found that watching TV affects children's eating behaviour in a number of ways. Children are more likely to eat unhealthy foods – more pizza, more sugary drinks, salty snacks and fewer fruits and vegetables – when they watch television. The research suggests that compared with children who never eat in front of the TV, children who do:

- Eat more in general.
- Eat more foods high in fat, salt and sugar.
- Eat less protein, fruit and vegetables.
- Are likely to be heavier.
- Make more unhealthy food choices.
- Make more requests for advertised foods.

One reason why children eat more when watching TV is probably because they are distracted – attention is drawn away from the food they are eating and is focused instead on following the action, making it easier to overeat. This is 'mindless eating' – adults do it too.

One famous experiment illustrates this nicely. Cinema-goers were given a medium or large bucket of 5-day-old popcorn to eat during a post-lunch matinee, i.e. when they were not hungry. Although the popcorn was very stale and presumably rather unpleasant, most participants ate it and those given the larger buckets ate even more. Seemingly, the participants were sufficiently distracted by the film that they didn't notice that the popcorn was past its best. In addition, eating popcorn while watching a film is a common habit and doing it frequently means that an association is formed between film-watching and eating which is very hard to break, even if what we are given to eat is not very nice! Children who habitually eat in front of the TV will not only eat more when they do so, but may learn to expect food every time the TV goes on.

Here are some useful tips to follow:

- Separate children's screen time from meals and snack time.

- Keep TV (and other screen media) out of your child's room.

- DVDs or channels without adverts are preferable.

- Watch specific programmes rather than just having the TV on.

Caitlin
mum of Tim (10), Lily (8) and George (4)

'My youngest watches around 3 to 4 hours per week of TV max. He has not been brought up in a culture of TV-watching, so it's not something he particularly enjoys or chooses to do. In terms of TV time he does have, we have made sure he has made a commitment to constructive watching – we do not "just" put on the TV – so he has chosen a particular sci-fi series and football matches (as he plays) each week. He watches 1 hour of his sci-fi show per week and 1 match per week (1.5 hours) and sometimes, ne and I watch an architectural show together, as he loves buildings.'

Children are exposed to advertising when watching TV

When was the last time you were watching TV with your little one and on came an advert for vegetables endorsed by a celebrity, or fruit being promoted by a well-loved cartoon character? Foods advertised on TV are predominantly high in fat, sugar and/or salt, and are processed foods such as confectionary, sugary breakfast cereals, sugary drinks and savoury snacks. Advertising of unprocessed foods such as fruit and vegetables, whole grains and fresh milk is virtually unheard of.

As will be discussed in Chapter 8, food advertising works. In one experiment, researchers found that children ate more food and specifically more unhealthy foods when they watched a TV advert for food than they did after watching the non-food ads.

TV increases liking for featured foods

Children prefer foods they have seen advertised on television to foods they have not. Given that the majority of food adverts targeted at children are for unhealthy high-fat, high-sugar, salty foods, the importance of limiting exposure to adverts is clear.

Product placement within TV shows and films can also affect children's likes and dislikes, and is used most often with sweetened drinks. In one experiment, half the children were shown a clip of a film in which a popular fizzy drink was featured, and the other half watched a section of the film without it. Children who had watched the clip with the drink in it were much more likely to ask for it than those who hadn't. This is advertising by stealth and is an effective and sneaky way around the rules for food manufacturers.

TV increases brand awareness and loyalty

Development of brand knowledge is important for food manufacturers since it is this awareness that drives children's requests for their product. For example, children are much more likely to ask for a branded cereal that they have seen advertised on television than a similar, supermarket own-brand cereal.

Research has shown that children as young as 18 months can recognise brands and by age 3 years, they have a much greater knowledge of unhealthy food brands than healthy brands. Some studies have even shown that children recognise brand logos before they can recognise their own name.

Brand knowledge increases significantly from age 3 to 4 years although children of this age are not capable of understanding the difference between advertisements that are selling products and normal TV content. This level of understanding doesn't develop until around the age of 8. As a result, many argue (rightly, in our view) that it is unethical to advertise to younger children in this way.

WHAT ARE THE REGULATIONS?

In 2010 the World Health Organization recommended that countries reduce exposure of children to marketing messages that 'promote foods high in saturated fats, trans-fatty acids, free sugars or salt, and to reduce the use of powerful techniques to market these foods to children'. However, recommendations are not legally binding and it is up to individual countries to legislate for themselves.

Countries differ in the extent to which they regulate junk-food advertising to children on television. The UK has some of the toughest regulations, having placed a ban on junk food advertising during programmes aimed at children (defined as under 16 years of age) or on specific children's channels. Product placement in children's programmes made in the UK, and the use of known cartoon characters, are also banned. However, there are still easily exploitable gaps in the legislation that you should be aware of.

'Family' programmes

The fact is that 71 per cent of children's viewing time is spent watching programmes that are not aimed specifically at children, but at the family as a whole.[17] Family programmes include family game shows, talent shows, sports, soap operas and family cartoons.

These are classified as 'adult' programmes and are therefore not covered by the regulations. The food industry capitalises on this by advertising unhealthy foods during these 'adult' programmes, and it has been reported that, despite the regulations, children's exposure to advertisements for junk foods has actually increased, albeit by a very small amount. Many believe

---

[17] stakeholders.ofcom.org.uk/binaries/broadcast/reviews-investigations/psb-review/psb2012/section-c.pdf

that there should be a watershed that prevents all advertising of foods and drinks before 9 p.m.

Other notable exceptions are:

- **Product placement** is banned in the UK, but the regulations do not apply to programming made outside the UK or to online advertising.

- **On-demand TV[18], radio advertising and mobile marketing[19]** are not covered by the regulations.

- **Programmes broadcast from unregulated countries** are also not covered.[20]

- **Cartoon characters owned by a particular company to advertise a product** are excluded from the legislation. Little research has been carried out on the impact of these 'brand equity characters' but a recent study of 4- to 8-year-old children suggested that children liked string-cheese products more when

---

[18] Choosing to watch a TV programme rather than a specific time when it is broadcast.

[19] Marketing through a mobile phone – usually a smartphone. This may be more personalised than TV adverts.

[20] Landon, 2013. News report. Gaps and weaknesses in controls on food and drink marketing to children in the UK. Appetite 62, p187-189

they were branded with a cartoon character than when they were not.

Of course television isn't the only medium through which advertisers can reach children, and the massive growth in Internet use has opened up an important new channel through which the food industry can target children.

ONLINE MARKETING AND 'ADVERGAMES'

The UK restrictions on advertising to children do not extend to brand promotion in online games and websites. Estimates suggest that 98 per cent of children's websites allow advertising[21] and two-thirds of websites for children rely on advertising as their main source of revenue.

Some manufacturers commission video games featuring their products, known as 'advergames'. Advergames are unregulated, and in the US an estimated 1.2million children are exposed to them. Rather than the passive viewing of a 30-second commercial in between TV shows, advergames engage children in the brand

---

[21] E. Neuborne, 'For Kids on the Web, It's an Ad, Ad, Ad, Ad World', Business Week 3475 (13 August 2001), 108–109

through play, meaning that children are exposed to more persistent and powerful advertising than when watching the TV.

Children are often given an electronic tablet to play with while out to dinner or as a treat for being good, so if you do this regularly it is a good idea to be savvy about the types of games children are playing on them, and to be aware that these might include advertising.

WHAT DOES THE SCIENCE SAY?

There is far less research on online marketing compared with that on TV. One experiment carried out in Portugal compared children's snack-food choices after they had played either an advergame advertising a healthy food or an unhealthy food. They found that children ate more unhealthy snack foods and fewer fruits and vegetables after playing unhealthy food advergames. However, where advergames promoted healthy foods, children were more likely to eat fruit and vegetables. [22] In reality the latter are few and far between.

Research suggests that children may be more vulnerable to online marketing since they recognise this as

---

[22] onlinelibrary.wiley.com/doi/10.1002/cb.359/abstract

advertising a lot later than they do with TV advertising. One study found that while 11- to 12-year-olds clearly understood that TV advertising was trying to sell a product to them, they were less able to recognise this in web advertising. It is likely that this difference arises from the fact that web advertising is embedded within the website, rather than separated from the programme as with TV advertising.[23]

MOBILE MARKETING

Though your child may still be too young to own a mobile phone, an increasing number of very young children do. In the UK, the use of mobile phones with internet access – 'smartphones' – is high, with 1 in 50 5- to 7-year-olds and 1 in 6 8- to 11-year-olds owning one.[24] Targeting children through their mobile phones is therefore another burgeoning avenue that the food industry is using to influence children. Using phones, children are able to browse the internet without parental control, and may be exposed to advertising not intended, and not suitable, for their age group.

---

[23] Blades, Oates, Li, 2012 Children's recognition of advertisements on television and on Web pages Appetite 63, p 90-93

[24] Children and parents: media use and attitudes. London, Ofcom, 2011 stakeholders.ofcom.org.uk/%20binaries/

Mobile marketing provides a cheap way for marketers to advertise their products, getting access to a large number of children any time they are online or using their mobile phone. Interactive websites and competitions permit the collection of mobile numbers and information on children's preferences. From this, marketers can use mobile messaging and can refine the advertising to products consistent with your child's preferences. Smartphones also provide a further avenue of access through apps, providing another opportunity for product placement.

TAKE-HOME MESSAGES

Promotion of products via advergames and mobile marketing is possible because of gaps in the regulations, providing a route for the food industry to target your child. The best means of defence is avoidance! Here are ways that you can keep your child safe:

- Ideally, under-2s should not watch any TV and try to limit over-2s to no more than 2 hours a day.

TAKE-HOME MESSAGES

- Try to separate children's screen time from meals and snack time, so no eating in front of the TV.

- Keep television, tablets and other screen media out of your child's room and monitor their use the rest of the time.

- Encourage your child to be active or creative – sports, arts, play – rather than watching TV or playing computer games.

- Be aware of the computer games your children are playing.

- Choose specific programmes or DVDs to watch rather than simply 'watching TV'.

- Avoid commercial channels where possible – CBBC has no advertising at all!

- Campaign for better regulations to protect your child. (See 'Resources and sources of further information' at the end of the book.)

CHAPTER EIGHT

The outside world:
food industry tactics

DESPITE THE FACT THAT children can and should eat the same good, healthy foods as adults, processed-food manufacturers have tried to convince us otherwise and there has been a massive increase in the availability of 'children's foods' in recent years. This chapter will help you to become a more informed, empowered and critical consumer by providing the facts about the food industry, the tactics they use to market foods to you and your child, and how these tactics make it harder to feed your children a healthy, balanced diet.

THE FOOD INDUSTRY: FACTS

The food industry is big business. We are bombarded with the choice of thousands of children's food products on the supermarket shelves, but the majority of these products, including the organic ones, are produced by just 10 multinational companies, who have annual sales of between $35 and $99 billion – more than the annual income of over 70 countries! These companies not only make food for your children, they make all kinds of products, from deodorants to washing powder, and slimming aids to bleach.

To maintain these sales figures, multinationals spend billions on marketing each year. In the US alone an estimated $1.79 billion (£1.04 billion) is spent on marketing food to children annually; only $280 million of this is on healthy food.[25] By 'the food industry' we are referring specifically to the 'processed'-food industry who, rather than selling simple, unprocessed fruit and vegetables or whole ingredients, manufacture processed children's foods which are cheaper, deliver higher margins and are therefore much more profitable than unprocessed foods like fruit and vegetables.

FOOD MARKETING TO PARENTS

As a parent, you are the gatekeeper of your children's food intake. However, the vast array of bewildering and sometimes contradictory nutritional messages on packaging and in advertising makes it difficult to know what really is healthy. Food manufacturers use a number of tactics to reassure and persuade you that their foods

---

[25] www.ftc.gov/sites/default/files/documents/reports/ review-food-marketing-children-and-adolescents-follow-report/121221foodmarketingreport.pdf

are vital for your child's health and well-being, with scant regard for the truth about their nutritional content. Here we describe some of these tactics:

Labelling

The European rules governing labelling are as follows:[26]

> 'The labelling, advertising and presentation of a food must not be such as could mislead a purchaser to a material degree particularly as to the characteristics of the food, and in particular as to its nature, identity, properties, composition, quantity, durability, origin or provenance, method of manufacture or production; by attributing to the food effects or properties that it does not possess; by suggesting the food possesses special characteristics when in fact all similar foods possess such characteristics.'

Although this appears to be fairly straightforward and clear, when targeting you as parents, manufacturers attempt to persuade you that their product is good for your child by using a variety of popular 'buzz' words. Below, we give a few examples that you should be aware of:

---

[26] Article 2 of Directive 2000/13/EC (on food labelling).

'Natural'

Foods can be labelled 'natural' as long as they do not contain added colour, artificial flavours or synthetic substances and are minimally processed. 'Natural' does *not* mean organic or healthy. Essentially, it means that the product is made from natural ingredients, e.g. ingredients 'produced by nature, not the work of man or interfered with by man',[27][28] although some processing in order to make the food fit for human consumption is permitted. Manufacturers have been known to take liberties with definitions of 'natural'. Recently a multi-million dollar lawsuit was settled with a major multinational for claiming their juices were 'natural' when in fact they contained synthetic vitamins, fibre and possibly genetically modified ingredients.

Almost all packaged foods are processed in some way in order to increase their shelf life, so very few are truly what we might consider 'natural'.

---

[27] Food Standards Agency www.food.gov.uk/northern-ireland/niregulation/niguidancenotes/fresh-pure-natural-ni

[28] Food and Drug Administration www.fda.gov/AboutFDA/Transparency/Basics/ucm214868.htm

'Organic'

EU/US standards state that if the label says '100 per cent organic' then it needs to contain 100 per cent organic ingredients. If the label states 'made from organic ingredients' then 70 per cent of the product must contain organic ingredients. Organic foods do not contain additives, preservatives, artificial sweeteners, colourings or flavourings, are usually free from genetically modified ingredients and are grown using more environmentally friendly agricultural practices than non-organic foods. In recent years it has become aspirational to feed children organic food, as our mothers elucidated:

Sue
mum of Peter (4) and Barney (17 months)

'Mum-and-baby groups, NCT etc., make you feel pressured into conforming to this "perfect mummy" role – where if the food isn't organic and lovingly picked and cuddled as it's prepared then you're a bad mother. (Sorry, I'm being v cynical here!)'

While the production of organic foods can be kinder to the environment, it is important to know that 'organic' does *not* necessarily mean healthy in terms of nutritional value, although organic foods are often promoted as a healthier version of the non-organic equivalent. As a health-conscious parent, you may be willing to pay more for organic foods, making them very lucrative products for the food industry:

Sally
mum of Daisy (3)

'I was sold by anything that said "organic"!!'

Alex
mum of Jack (2.5)

'I liked the idea that he was eating organic meat/ fish. However, I am not convinced it made too much difference overall. I suppose it feels as though the food is slightly better quality which is reassuring.'

However, there is no scientific consensus that organic foods are any healthier than their non-organic counterparts. Two reviews examining over 200 scientific articles found no difference between the nutritional content of organic and conventional foods, nor any health benefits.

Organic does *not* mean fair trade. Organic also does *not* mean unprocessed: the shelf-life of organic, processed foods are often similar to regular foods, so they will have been processed as much as regular foods too. Furthermore, you can buy many organic children's foods that have been processed so much that they look nothing like real food at all!

'A source of . . .' or 'Fortified with . . .'

The labels on many children's foods state that the product is a good source of a particular nutrient or is fortified with vitamins and minerals. The effect of this is twofold: it reassures you that the product is healthy, but the intention is also to distract you from noticing other, less desirable, ingredients in the product, such as excess sugar.

There is a perception that the more nutrients in a product the better, so labels often say things like: 'Provides at least 100 per cent of vitamin D.' However, scientific studies show that giving *healthy* children extra nutrients has no added health benefits (and may actually be toxic and bad for their health in the longer term). One review of vitamin D supplementation, for example, found no improvement in bone density in healthy children with normal vitamin D levels.

Labelling a product as a '*source of* iron, vitamins and minerals' does not necessarily mean that the product is really nutritious, since it may only contain a trace of the nutrients required as part of a balanced diet.

Why do products need to be fortified? To increase the shelf life of packaged children's foods, manufacturers must heat it for a long time to kill bacteria, but good nutrients may be destroyed in the process, so manufacturers fortify them with artificial vitamins and minerals. While fortified products are better than their non-fortified equivalents, there is the potential for some of these nutrients to be 'overconsumed'. Furthermore, there is not enough evidence about the potential risks of this over a long period of time.

Unfortunately, *unprocessed* foods do not come with labels extolling their virtues, but it's worth knowing that beef, apricots and chickpeas are all good sources of iron, and oily fish and sunlight[29] provide vitamin D, with none of the nasties! Nor can they be 'overconsumed' like their artificial counterparts.

'Mum's own recipe' or 'Mum's number-one choice'

Meaningless! These labels on children's food are designed to appeal to parents' sense that home-made food is best and are an attempt to persuade them that the products are pretty much the same as 'home-made', using 'the same kind of ingredients you have at home'. However, given what we now know about the intense heating of ingredients to improve shelf life, these foods are not like any home-made food you are likely to make!

'Healthy'

These foods may be anything but healthy. They do have to meet guidelines for fat, cholesterol and salt but they can contain a lot of sugar, preservatives and artificial ingredients.

---

[29] A few minutes a day in sunlight are sufficient for our bodies to make enough vitamin D. (It is less than the time that is needed for the skin to burn, but remember to enjoy sunlight safely and stay out of midday sun.)

'Made with wholegrain' or 'multigrain'

'Wholegrain' means the entire grain seed exists in its original form. 100% of the original kernel – all of the bran, germ, and endosperm – must be present to qualify as a whole grain[30]. 'Multigrain' just means that there are a number of grains, not necessarily that any of them are whole grains. If the label states 'made with wholewheat' or 'multigrain', then they probably only contain a small amount. Wholegrain products are marketed as healthy products; however, these products are only 100 per cent whole grain or whole wheat if the label actually says this. Processing of grains often removes their useful nutrients – so that again artificial fortification is needed.

'No added sugar, preservatives or flavourings'

Products that are labelled as having no added sugars, preservatives or artificial flavourings may be those that would not normally have contained these anyway. They may also contain fruit or fruit juice as sweeteners. These are also sugars, albeit in a different, apparently more healthy form.

---

[30] wholegrainscouncil.org/whole-grains-101/definition-of-whole-grains

Misleading names and pictures

To maximise profits, manufacturers often bulk out foods with cheap ingredients such as water, and thickening agents such as refined rice, corn or wheat flours. Processing food in this way reduces the nutrients in the products but increases the volume. So as well as the use of persuasive language, manufacturers may use misleading pictures to convince you of the integrity and healthiness of their products. Labels may show pictures of wholesome foods, fresh vegetables, healthy cows and happy babies. However, when you look more closely at the product's ingredients, they may not contain the quantities of fresh grains, vegetables and meats implied by the pictures on the packaging.

The few regulations that exist about the wording on labels are often ambiguous and manufacturers use this ambiguity to their advantage. For example, EU regulations state that if a protein comes first when listed on the label then the product must be made up of at least 10 per cent of that protein. Manufacturers have to move the protein down the order of ingredients on the label, but you can still be misled into expecting a higher protein content than is actually provided.

Another regulation states that if just one ingredient

is featured in the name of the dish, it should contain at least 40 per cent of that ingredient. However, this regulation does not appear to be enforced when it comes to 'one-pot dishes', where the main ingredient is meat. There are examples of well-known brands where the dish only contains 8 per cent of the main meat ingredient, and others contain as little as 5 per cent. Most contain far less than 40 per cent meat.

Appealing to the 'sweet tooth'

Chapter 3 explained the necessity of providing children early on with a range of different tastes – especially more bitter tastes such as green vegetables. It is somewhat surprising then that there are so few vegetable purées for weaning on the market, and that those that do exist are purées of sweet vegetables e.g. carrot and sweet potato, rather than the more bitter, green varieties. As described in chapter 3, some products do exist that contain a mix of green vegetables, but often these are sweetened with fruits, creating some very odd combinations. For example, varieties currently available include: 'Pears, peas and broccoli', 'Apples, green beans and raisins', 'Kale, apple and Greek yoghurt' and 'Broccoli and apple'. We could go on, but would really rather not!

The problem is that children eating these odd flavour combinations will not get used to the taste of real vegetables and rapidly start to expect everything to be sweet. Why manufacturers produce these instead of more normal combinations or, indeed, single flavours is unclear, but may have something to do with the fact that parents themselves may doubt that their child would like less sweet vegetable dishes and therefore wouldn't buy them. Again, as we discussed in Chapter 3, infants are particularly open to new tastes, will eat and enjoy all sorts of more 'grown-up' flavours and should be encouraged to do so. When considering buying these combination foods, ask yourself whether you might make such a dish for yourself to eat and, if not, then consider buying something else.

Aspirational packaging

As with any product, manufacturers are always looking for a new angle. In the baby-food world, 'pouch foods' are an example of a currently 'in vogue' product.

Sally
mum of Daisy (3)

'I used 2 main brands mainly. Loved the squeeze packs for convenience. Also had a shop nearby that sold all-natural apple purée with other mixtures of fruit, which were great and very popular!'

These pouches were invented by an organic baby food company and therefore retain a healthy, aspirational aura. In addition, they are convenient and mess-free as children can simply drink the contents. While we fully understand this need for convenience, and that using these products from time to time does not harm your child, there are a number of facts about pouches that you may want to consider. Chapter 3 has more information on this issue.

FOOD MARKETING TO CHILDREN

While there are stringent government regulations ensuring the safety of children's foods, there are few regulations in the marketing of these products. For example, there are no regulations concerning:

- The use of brand-owned cartoon characters on packaging and labelling of high fat, sugar and salt.
- The presence of vending machines full of crisps and sweets in public leisure centres.
- Marketing in schools, for example through branded school equipment.
- The advertising of products in stores.
- The practice of free giveaways such as a toy with a meal.

As we've described, children become targets of food advertising, and research shows that manufacturers aggressively market their most unhealthy products to children. In Chapter 7 we discussed the use of television and screen media advertising, but there are many other ways in which the food industry market their products. The use of cartoon characters and celebrity endorsers on packaging, product placement in supermarkets, competitions, free toys – all are used to market food directly to children. Unethical as they may be, these techniques remain relatively unregulated. Marketing food in this way undermines your efforts to get your children to eat healthily and increases the likelihood of your child pestering you to buy these products.

Appealing packaging and giveaways

Manufacturers make food look appealing to children by using brightly coloured packaging, often featuring cartoon characters and often including some free item.

Amy
mum of Eva (4)

'Advertising of unhealthy food is very prominent and colourful and often offers free stickers or a kit to make a dinosaur or something that draws kids in. They also use popular characters as drawing-in points, especially on drinks (the sugary ones) and Eva just automatically wants that one, not for the taste factor but for who is on the bottle. It's really hard to say no and say you can have this other one . . . I have had some battles, but I do sometimes give in.'

Research shows that this not only influences the foods that children ask for but also what they are willing to eat. For example, one study from the US found that 50 per cent of children say that food from a package featuring a cartoon tastes better than exactly the same food from a plain package. A survey of 2,000 parents found that using cartoons in this way makes shopping more stressful because they have to keep saying no to their children.[31]

The case of breakfast cereals

Breakfast cereals are the products most heavily marketed to children and are taken as an example here. For parents, packaged cereals are quick and easy, children like them and eat them, they are served with nutritious milk and the packaging usually reassures parents that they are full of lots of vitamins and minerals. So what is the problem?

High levels of sugar

Guidelines suggest that a 100 g portion of cereal should contain no more than 5 g of added sugar, yet many cereals contain more than 20 g per 100 g – 4 times more than is recommended. Some contain as much as 6 times more than the recommended level of sugar at 30 g per 100 g of cereal – more than some chocolate biscuits![32] Even those cereals often

[31] Which? Campaign report. Shark Tales and Incredible Endorsements www.which.co.uk/documents/pdf/shark-tales-and-incredible-endorsements-which-report-176879.pdf

[32] www.actiononsalt.org.uk/news/Salt%20in%20the%20news/2012/64061.html

marketed as healthy or natural, contain considerable quantities of sugar. It is probably no surprise then that breakfast cereals are the second biggest contributor to children's daily sugar intake in the UK (after sugary drinks). One US study reported that children who eat cereal every day for breakfast will consume more than 4.5 kg of sugar a year.

Low levels of nutrients

Cereals are not just high in sugar but also generally low in natural nutrients because of the harsh processing required to turn grains into the finished product – puffed or crunchy flakes. They are therefore (re) 'fortified with iron' or 'vitamin enriched'.

If the use of cartoons influences the foods children are willing to eat, then perhaps they might be better used to promote fruit and vegetables. However, there is very little research in this area. In one notable exception, some 4- to 5-year-old children were given small containers of fresh fruit or vegetables, each with a picture of a well-known cartoon character on it. The researchers found that these children ate more of the fruit and vegetables than children who were given plain containers of fruit and vegetables.[33] While this was a small study, it does suggest that using cartoons to advertise healthy foods could be beneficial. Making healthy food fun is highly effective – think back to one mum's description of homemade 'Mr and Mrs Pizza faces' back in Chapter 4.

Links with sport

Sponsorship

Sports events ought to be a good place to promote healthy eating, and yet sponsorship of sporting events is often dominated by manufacturers of unhealthy food and drinks – a lost opportunity for health promotion.

In sponsoring sports events, the food industry's motive is twofold:

- It allows them to advertise to children through television, since sports programmes are not included in the regulations. This creates brand association, which provides an illusion of healthiness for their product.

- Their associations with sporting events suggest to

---

[33] www.ncbi.nlm.nih.gov/pubmed/?term=keller+vegetable+children+package

people that as long as you are physically active you are healthy, which is not strictly true.

In addition to sponsoring sports events and matches, there is a proliferation of food companies involved in sponsorship of community activities. For example, a well-known chocolate manufacturer sponsors physical activity programmes for children, while another sponsors community football facilities.

Sporting celebrity endorsement

Sporting celebrities are often employed to promote unhealthy children's foods. One study from the US found that 102 food products in just 2 supermarkets were endorsed by a sports person or contained pictures of a character exercising. Many of these were unhealthy foods or sugar-sweetened drinks targeted at children.

The impact of the 'endorser effect' was highlighted in a novel experiment from the UK whereby 8- to 11-year-olds were asked to watch a television ad for either: 1) a specific brand of crisps, featuring a celebrity sportsman; 2) a savoury food with no celebrity; 3) TV footage of the same celebrity but in a TV-presenter role; or 4) a commercial for a non-food item. They were then offered crisps to eat. They found that children who had viewed (1) or (3) ate more of the crisps compared with children who watched (2) or (4).

Unhealthy foods in sporting facilities
Even when children are actively participating in sports they are exposed to junk foods, since many sports facilities permit the installation of vending machines full of unhealthy snacks and sweets. In one study in Canada, recreational facility managers were interviewed and reported that financial constraints were the biggest barrier to selling healthier foods in vending machines, as they believed that they would be less profitable than junk foods. In one study conducted in Australia, 77 per cent of children were found to participate every week in organised sport sponsored by food companies – in particular rugby and cricket. It comes as no surprise then, that unhealthy foods are the only foods available at most sports stadia. Many parents have reported frustration at this:

'The thing is . . . if you're taking children to the game with you . . . there's nothing there for them – there wouldn't be anything healthy for you to buy a child at all.'[34]

---

[34] Reproduced from: R Ireland and F Watkins, 'Football fans and food: a case study of a football club in the English Premier League' Public Health Nutrition 2010 13, 682–687, with permission from lead author.

The European Healthy Stadia Network is working hard to make sports stadia across Europe become more health-promoting environments. One innovative programme from this network is the 'Healthy Stadia Catering Mark', which aims to help sports clubs provide healthier menus during events. (To find out more, check out the 'Resources and sources of further information' section.)

Product placement in supermarkets

Manufacturers pay for products to be placed at child's eye level on the supermarket shelf to attract their attention, and this is successful in increasing sales. Industry studies suggest parents spend 10–40 per cent more whilst shopping if their children are with them!

Many supermarkets also put high-fat, high-sugar confectionary at the checkout in order to catch you at your weakest – you've made it around the supermarket without giving in to requests for all sorts of undesirable foods, you are unloading the trolley with a queue of grumpy shoppers behind you, and suddenly your child has grabbed a packet of sweets and is crying to be allowed to have them. The frequency of scenes like this and the negative reaction to this type of product placement is possibly why some UK supermarkets (although not all) have agreed to stop selling confectionary at the main checkouts.

Food manufacturers and advertisers use the sorts of tactics we have discussed because they work to increase desire for their products in your child. The more aware you are of what they are trying to do, the better you will be able to avoid the pitfalls. Legislation to curtail less than 100 per cent ethical practices is not on the cards any time soon and the industry has not, to date, shown that it is very good at regulating itself. Be an informed and critical consumer when shopping with, and for, your child and demand that your supermarkets and sports clubs stay on message about healthy eating!

EATING OUT

It's always a treat to eat out – to have someone else cook for you every now and then – but for children, eating out can be a chore since they have to sit still for longer than usual, and eat when they would rather play. The frequency of eating out has increased in the past decades (in the UK it now accounts for 11 per cent of daily energy intake; in the US it accounts for 16 per cent of children's or adolescents' energy intake) and for some families it has become an almost daily activity, rather than an infrequent treat. This can be problematic since children's menus rarely contain healthy options.

One study in the US analysed a vast number of children's menus and found that just 12 out of 3,039 children's meal options met nutritional standards for pre-school-aged children and only 15 met nutritional standards for older children. Some snacks on offer contained as many as 1,500 calories (almost a whole day's energy requirement!).

Children who regularly eat fast food consume more calories, fat, sugar and sugary drinks, and less fruit, vegetables and fibre than children who do not. In the US, a third of children and adolescents consume fast food each day. A survey of the food on offer for children in UK restaurants found that:

- 8 out of 21 restaurants studied did not have any vegetables or salad in their children's menu.

- 11 out of 21 did not have any fruit as dessert.

- 12 out of 21 had children's menus comprising only chicken nuggets, burgers and sausages.

- Some children's fast-food meals contained far more than the recommended 4 g of salt a day.

The researchers conducting the survey found that 66 per cent of parents thought that food provision in restaurants was not good enough. Menus generally do not contain nutritional information, making it impossible for parents to know how much salt, saturated fat and sugar their child is consuming when eating out. Furthermore, only 1 restaurant in the study (a Jamie's Italian restaurant) could say where their meat had come from.

Fiona
mum of Harry (18 months)

'I find that children's menus are too old for my 18-month-old, or contain foods with too much salt. For instance – sausage, mash and gravy. I would never serve my child gravy because of the salt content of it.'

Major fast-food outlets market heavily towards children, with children's meals featuring cartoon characters and free toy giveaways. In the US, $360 million was spent on toys to be distributed with children's meals in 2007,[36] but there is some good practice out there: some

---

[36] www.rwjf.org/content/dam/farm/reports/reports/2010/rwjf68794

restaurants are beginning to offer smaller portions of healthier adult options, while others offer a healthier children's menu. This mum explains how she deals with the problems of eating out with small children:

Penny
mum of Poppy (6) and Stan (2)

'If I can see that the restaurant has certain ingredients, I'll ask them to make something with them even if it isn't on the menu. Often we will have a selection of food, some from the starter section, some from the sides, and some from the mains and just have it all together. When Poppy was being picky I'd just ask for plain things, like a burger and a bun with no sauce or salad or anything.'

Don't be afraid to be assertive about what you want for your child. Restaurants will only change if we tell them what we want them to do.

TAKE-HOME MESSAGES

We hope this chapter has given you some insights into how the food industry operates, and we leave it here with a summary and some tips to help you to deal with some of the negative impacts of their marketing practices:

- The food industry uses a variety of techniques to market 'children's' food that is high in fat, sugar and salt.

- Be a critical consumer – be aware of their tactics.

- Words and pictures on food labels can be misleading.

- Buy foods for your child that you would eat yourself – healthy foods for adults can be healthy foods for children too.

- Avoid odd food combinations in baby foods and avoid savoury dishes that are sweetened with added sugars or fruits.

- Supermarkets and restaurants act on customer demand – be a demanding consumer and ask for better!

CHAPTER NINE

Happy ever after

OUR AIM IN THIS book was to bring the findings of scientific research into children's eating behaviour to a wider and more relevant audience – the parents and carers of young children. You are the ones on the front line, trying to deal with the idiosyncratic eating habits of your children, whilst simultaneously fighting off the advances of the processed-food industry.

We hope we have provided interesting reading as well as practical help and that you will feel empowered to try some of the techniques we suggest. We would like to send you away with our top tips for stress-free feeding. Tradition would dictate that there are 10, but there's no getting away from it – we have 11!

Here goes:

One

From pregnancy onwards, eat the healthy foods that you most want your child to enjoy and be enthusiastic about the taste. Keep your dislikes to yourself!

Two

Breastfeed if you can and for as long as possible, BUT don't beat yourself up if it doesn't work for your and your baby. However you feed your baby, just try to be close and cuddly while feeding, and make lots of eye contact.

Three

From birth, respect your child's ability to tell when she is full. Never insist that a bottle is finished or a plate cleared.

Four

Offer a wide variety of vegetables as first weaning foods and not just the sweeter ones (carrots, sweet potatoes). Go crazy and give spinach or broccoli as well!

Five

If your 5-month-old baby is snatching the food off your plate and chomping on it, it might be time to begin introducing solid food. Don't leave it till too long after 6 months with a normally developing infant.

Six

When offering unfamiliar foods, ignore facial expressions of apparent dislike. Ask yourself, Is she happily eating it? If the answer is yes, forget the face!

Seven

Offer new foods lots of times before giving up. Repeated tasting is by far the most effective way of changing food preferences. It may take as many as 15 tastings to work. Give lots of praise, encouragement and a sticker for each tasting if it helps.

Eight

Keep lots of fruit and vegetables in the house and avoid bringing fatty and sugary stuff into the house at all. Your child knows about the sweets you 'hide' on the top shelf and wants them even more because they are forbidden.

Nine

Relax about grandparents spoiling your toddler with unhealthy treats unless it is a daily problem. Try to negotiate, but if you don't succeed in persuading them to stop, be clear and firm with your child that what happens with Granny does not happen at home!

Ten

Watching TV, especially when eating, should be limited in terms of *what* they watch and for *how long*.

Eleven

Food manufacturers and supermarkets will try anything legal (or even illegal, if they think they can get away with it) to sell their products to you and your child. Complain about bad practice.

And finally, here is a reminder of the products and practices to avoid:

Follow-on milks, growing-up milks and similar: You don't need these. Breast milk and first formula milk are fine until 12 months, and then give full-fat cow's milk.

Sugary milkshakes for fussy eaters: High calorie and full of sugar, these will fill up your child leaving them with no appetite to try healthy foods.

'Children's foods': Children are just small humans – they don't need special food or snacks. Sometimes these foods don't even look like food. If you wouldn't eat it yourself, don't offer it to your child!

Avoid rewarding, distracting or comforting with food: Help your child to develop a healthy relationship with food; to learn that food is simply a delicious solution to feeling hungry, not a cure for sadness or boredom.

Try to stay calm: It's tough sometimes, but keeping your cool will pay off in happier, healthier mealtimes for the whole family.

GOOD LUCK!

Resources and sources of further information

GENERAL INFORMATION:

Mumsnet: www.mumsnet.com
Netmums: www.netmums.com
Change4Life: www.nhs.uk/change4life
Start4Life: www.nhs.uk/start4life
National Institute of Clinical Excellence: www.nice.org.uk
Children's Food Trust: www.childrensfoodtrust.org.uk

THE EARLY YEARS: MILK FEEDING

Unicef/NHS: www.unicef.org.uk
Unicef UK, the Baby Friendly Initiative: www.babyfriendly.org.uk
Association of Breastfeeding Mothers: www.abm.me.uk
La Leche League: www.laleche.org.uk
Best Beginnings: www.bestbeginnings.org.uk
National Childbirth Trust: www.nct.org.uk
Start4Life: www.nhs.uk/start4life
First Steps Nutrition Trust: www.firststepsnutrition.org
Baby Milk Action: www.babymilkaction.org

WEANING

Baby-led weaning, further information: www.babyledweaning.com
Judy More, *Stress-free Weaning* (Hodder Education, 2010)

FUSSY EATING

Tiny Tastes packs to help parents manage fussy eating: www.
weightconcern.org.uk/tinytastes

Child feeding guide for fussy eaters:
www.childfeedingguide.co.uk

GRANDPARENTS AND OTHER CHILDCARE

Family and Childcare Trust: www.familyandchildcaretrust.org
Grandparents Plus: www.grandparentsplus.org.uk
The Grandparents' Association: www.grandparents-association.
org.uk
Grannynet: www.grannynet.co.uk
Gransnet: www.gransnet.com

VITAMINS AND MINERALS

NHS: www.nhs.uk
Vitamin D guidance:
www.nice.org.uk/guidance/indevelopment/GID-PHG71

CHILDHOOD OVERWEIGHT AND OBESITY

Weight Concern: www.weightconcern.org.uk

SCREEN TIME

Parent Port: www.parentport.org.uk
Advertising Standards Agency: www.asa.org.uk

FOOD MARKETING

Sustain: www.sustainweb.org/
British Heart Foundation: www.bhf.org.uk
Which? Consumer advice: www.which.co.uk
Children's food campaign:
www.sustainweb.org/childrensfoodcampaign
Marion Nestle, *Food Politics: How the Food Industry Influences
Nutrition and Health* (University of California Press, 2002)

HEALTHY EATING AND SPORTS

The European Healthy Stadia Network: www.healthystadia.eu